THE
SEVENTH-DAY DIET

THE SEVENTH-DAY DIET

How the "Healthiest People in America" Live Better, Longer, Slimmer—And How You Can Too

Chris Rucker *and* Jan Hoffman

RANDOM HOUSE
New York

This book is not intended as a substitute for the medical advice of physicians. The reader should regularly consult his doctor in matters relating to health and particularly in respect to symptoms that may require diagnosis or medical attention.

Various figures and tables in this work are derived or adapted from *Six Extra Years* by Lewis R. Walton, Jo Ellen Walton, and John A. Scharffenberg, published by Woodbridge Press, Santa Barbara, California 93160.

Library of Congress Cataloging-in-Publication Data

Rucker, Chris
The Seventh-Day diet: how the "healthiest people in America" live better, longer, slimmer—and how you can too/by Chris Rucker and Jan Hoffman.
p.   cm.
Includes bibliographical references and index.
ISBN 0-394-58473-2
1. Reducing diets.   2. Health.   I. Hoffman, Jan.   II. Title.
RM222.2.H574   1991
613.2′5—dc20   90-53488

Manufactured in the United States of America

98765432

First Edition

Designed by Virginia Tan

To Mackie, Krisha, and Aaron, who love the delicious, wholesome foods they were raised on; to Kelly, who has grown to like steamed vegetables and nut sauces; and to Kate, who has learned to eat potatoes and carrots.

A Word About Seventh-Day Adventists

We would like to stress that Seventh-Day Adventists are not a monolithic group, all of whom think and live exactly alike. In fact, not all Adventists are vegetarians (a circumstance that has made possible many studies on the differences between the health of vegetarians and nonvegetarians).

However, it is fair to say that most Seventh-Day Adventists have a commitment to a healthful life-style—thus their status as the "healthiest people in America." It is not the purpose of this book to explore the variations in levels of commitment to this life-style among Adventists, but to present principles of the Adventist life-style in general and workable terms so that others may incorporate features of it into their own lives.

Acknowledgments

Preparing this book was a heart-and-soul experience for me. Whatever I have accomplished has been thanks to the effort, prayers, and wise counsel of some very dedicated individuals to whom I am truly grateful. Thanks especially to my precious husband and children, who have provided loving support and a creative environment in which to prepare this book; to Dr. John Scharffenberg, who has always encouraged me and has supplied much-needed research; to the church I love, which has dramatically impacted my life and given me a foundation in health education; and finally and most gratefully, to my God, who has been my Ebenezer, my "stone of help," who has graciously made it all possible. —C.R.

I would like to thank my children and my fiancé for their tolerance and good humor during the year it took to write this book; Janet Kilby for much of the information in Chapter 6; and the staff at the Vanderbilt Medical Center Library for their invaluable help. —J.H.

Foreword

This book describes well the Adventist thinking on good nutrition. It also delineates present scientific thinking on diet, exercise, and health.

Two-thirds of the population in Western industrialized countries now die from just two causes—cardiovascular diseases and cancer. These are due primarily to the same two factors—cigarette smoking and bad diet. There are in turn three major factors that contribute to these ailments: too much fat (especially animal fat) in the diet, a lack of fiber, and obesity.

If the problem of fat, especially the animal fat, were taken care of, there would be little obesity. And getting the fat problem under control would solve the fiber problem: A low-fat diet results automatically in a high-fiber diet and a high-fat diet results automatically in a low-fiber diet.

This book does an excellent job of showing how to handle all these problems in a very practical and palatable way.

Adventists were leading the way in good nutrition a hundred years before scientists began to echo them. Ellen G. White, an Adventist leader considered to be a messenger with special light from the Lord, constantly pointed to the Bible as the source of good information on nutrition and health. She advocated the diet described in Genesis 1 and 3—fruits, whole grains, vegetables, nuts, and seeds—eaten at proper times ("Eat in due season," Eccl. 12:17) and in proper amounts ("Beware of surfeiting and drunkenness," Luke 21:34, Deut. 21:18–21). Alcohol (Prov. 20:1), unclean meats (Lev. 11; Deut. 14, Isa. 65 and 66), the fat of meat (Lev. 3:17), and other harmful things were forbidden.

No wonder Adventists live longer than most—the Bible had all the answers. However, the Bible is not just for Adventists, and the health principles it contains are for everyone, religious or not. Those who heed the advice contained in this book will be assured a better life. If you have a weight problem, you will find abundant help here, but these are good principles for anyone who wishes to be in the best of health. As a student of nutrition I recommend that you start on the program now.

—John A. Scharffenberg,
M.D., M.P.H. Adjunct Professor of Nutrition,
Loma Linda University, Loma Linda, CA,
and Medical Director, Pacific Health Education Center,
Bakersfield, CA

Contents

Introduction

Early in 1989 I signed up for Chris Rucker's nine-week weight-loss and healthy-living class. I was a little stubborn about learning anything new about health and nutrition (I thought I knew all I needed to know!), but the twelve extra pounds I was carrying around were stubborn, too, and I was willing to listen to a few lectures if it would help me fit into my favorite clothes again.

I had heard that Chris knew a way to lose weight that did not involve keeping a nervous eye on calories and portions at every meal. Constant calorie-watching was my way of losing weight, and it always worked. But every time I relaxed my vigil, the pounds came creeping back!

An experienced dieter such as I am has lost weight many times. I was tired of doing it alone.

Chris is accustomed to teaching classes in hospitals and corporations to groups of fifty to a hundred or more. Our group, a small one, met in a vegetarian restaurant after hours each Tuesday evening.

Slim, energetic Chris spoke for more than an hour the first night. She told us her program was much more than a diet—it was a way of life. Chris spoke of the benefits of daily brisk walks, drinking lots of water, and eating whole grains, and of the dangers of sugar, cholesterol, and saturated fat. This was information I had heard before, and I had used some of it in my own life, but I began to pay closer attention when I realized Chris had a complete vision of what a healthy life-style could be. She had an understanding of how the elements of a healthful diet can all work together. She had worked out many of the problems that people encounter when they make a decision to lose weight, or take better care of their bodies, or both. Being healthy began to sound workable and fun.

Chris spoke of the serious health problems that undermine the happiness of many Americans. I knew there were good reasons to improve one's diet other than the loss of a few pounds. I knew that cancer and heart disease were considered to be "epidemic" in America. As Chris gave us some statistics concerning these and other degenerative diseases, I began to think of the families I knew who had suffered or were suffering because of them. There is strong evidence that a large percentage of the degenerative diseases is linked not only to smoking and excessive drinking, but to unsound nutrition.

Chris's style was positive and encouraging. She wanted to help us realize the benefits of living healthfully, but she did not want to goad us with guilt or give us a diet that was more punishment than pleasure. She simply wanted to tell us all she could about health and nutrition, to encourage us in each healthful step we were able to take, and to answer our questions as difficulties arose. In addition to that, she had created some marvelous recipes that I was soon to discover were hearty and full of flavor and were relatively simple to prepare. She told us we would learn how to make waffles, gravies, desserts, and other fun foods that would make children want to be included in a healthful eating plan.

When she told us we would not have to count calories and that we could enjoy real meals and eat till we were satisfied, I wanted to stand up and cheer! Eating to satisfy an appetite is an experience that I and many other weight-conscious people sometimes fear has been lost to us forever. Chris told us that it would be helpful to pay attention to portions in the very beginning—but that in most cases this would simply be to ensure that we ate *enough* food! The key to losing weight while eating satisfying meals would be found in the kinds of foods eaten, and the number and distribution of meals. We learned that it is not necessary to count calories—but that calories do count! The reason it is not necessary to count calories is that when the basic health principles are followed, calories are automatically reduced.

Shortly after that first class I learned about a group of people (of which Chris herself is a member) that follows the basic health principles we would learn and that lives right here in America. In this land of affluent living, stressful daily schedules, high-fat diets, and the tragic diseases that often result, this group of people have managed to beat the odds. They are the Seventh-Day Adventists.

I had heard of Seventh-Day Adventism simply because Seventh-Day Adventists have been the subjects of an incredible amount of scientific research. Researchers in the health field take a strong interest in them, in part because Seventh-Day Adventists are generally acknowledged to be *the healthiest group of people living in America today*.

A few statistics will illustrate the strength of this claim:

• Male Seventh-Day Adventists have an 8.9-year longer average life expectancy than does the general population, while female members have a 7.5-year longer average life expectancy. These statistics include *all* Seventh-Day Adventists, even those who follow the health principles only loosely. It is thought that a life expectancy study done on those Adventists who follow the health principles consistently would yield even more dramatic results.

• Though it is not completely certain why this is so, vegetarian Seventh-Day Adventists have a reduced risk of osteoporosis when compared to meat-eaters in the general population. This probably has something to do with the fact that the excess protein in a high-meat diet causes the excretion of calcium in the urine. The SDA diet is both richer in calcium and lower in protein than the average American diet.

• Seventh-Day Adventists have a lower incidence of breast, prostate, pancreatic, bladder, and ovarian cancers than does the general population. Vegetarian Seventh-Day Adventists are *one-half* as likely as people in the general population to get colon or rectal cancer.

• Nonvegetarian male Adventists have 56 percent of the expected coronary heart disease mortality. (This means the rate of heart disease in these Adventists is 56 percent of the rate in the general American population). The heart disease mortality rate for lacto-ovo vegetarian men is 39 percent, while vegetarian male Adventists who use no meat, milk or eggs (total vegetarians) have an expected coronary heart disease mortality rate that is only 12 percent of that of the general population!

• Seventh-Day Adventists do not believe that "aches and pains" are an inevitable part of the aging process, nor do they believe that senility or deterioration of mental faculties are inevitable. They believe the mind should actually gain in range and power as one grows older.

Through their churches, schools, and publications, as well as through their hospitals, wellness centers, clinics, community service centers, and restaurants, Seventh-Day Adventists teach prevention of disease by life-style management. Their aim is to help others discover the quality of life they were designed to have.

Throughout this book you will find references to the writings of a woman named Ellen G. White, a Seventh-Day Adventist pioneer who lived and wrote in New England from the mid-1800s to the turn of the century. When she died she left behind a large body of writings, much of it on health and nutrition. Her ideas on health seem remarkable to us today because they predate much of the nutritional knowledge that has been uncovered by scientists only in the last few decades. As one writer has noted, what is perhaps most striking about White's thinking on the subject is

> her insistence on a well-balanced diet, before the phrase was even invented; her emphasis on natural foods in season whenever possible, long before anyone was aware of the destructive effects of preservation; her denunciation of meat, especially animal fat, a century before "cholesterol" and "polyunsaturated" found their way into dictionaries; and her rejection of refined foods, particularly flour and sugar, before scientists even suspected there were such things as "vitamins" that could be destroyed in the refining process.

To this day, Seventh-Day Adventists respect Ellen G. White's writings that constantly point to biblical principles of health and have benefited dramatically from following her nutritional advice.

What does this mean for those of us who are not Seventh-Day Adventists? It means that instead of waiting for science to give us a "magic pill" for cancer, instead of waiting for more expensive, sophisticated types of surgery to control heart disease, instead of cringing at the thought of another painful, self-depriving weight-loss program, we can take a look at the practices of a people who have found a better way. Scientists in the field of nutrition tell us that new research may at any moment change our ideas of what "perfect nutrition" is. Does this mean we are to wait for more research so we can find out what we should eat? For now, it might be more useful to take a look at the healthiest people in America and find out what *they* eat!

There are many reasons for pursuing good health: more years and better quality time to spend with your family, greater productivity and enjoyment of work, the ability to enjoy sports and other activities longer—and the capacity to just plain feel good! And there's certainly nothing *wrong* with the clear skin, shiny hair, and slim, strong bodies that naturally result from following the SDA principles!

Every Tuesday night I continued to go to class, received handouts and recipes for the week, stepped on the scales—smiled—and sat down to listen to Chris's encouraging advice. Sometimes she included a cooking demonstration or a film. Always, before she began to speak, she encouraged class members to share the problems and successes we had experienced with the program during the week. If a person had lost weight—even a half-pound—or taken some other important step, Chris led the group in a round of applause.

On the final Tuesday there was no lecture. Each person brought a dish prepared from the collection of recipes that Chris had created for us. There was a tasty punch, smooth and cool and fruity. Chris had made Veggie Spaghetticini, a lovely pasta-and-vegetable dish. There was a Zucchini Quiche, with a thick, flavorful filling and a whole-wheat crust made without lard or hydrogenated shortening that was—no kidding—really flaky. I brought a plate of steamed broccoli and cauliflower topped with Chris's creamy Pimiento Cashew Cheese sauce, which is made, astonishingly, without any cheese at all but uses instead a combination of fresh natural ingredients that some people find they actually prefer to real cheese! For dessert there was an apple pie that was so sweetly spiced I could not remember ever having had better.

By this time I was growing to prefer wholesome food to "the other kind," and I was feeling better than I had in a long time.

And in nine weeks I had lost ten pounds.

I would like you to have the opportunity to attend Chris's classes through the pages of this book. The first seven chapters are arranged according to the seven health principles that were presented to us week by week. We encourage you to absorb them at your own pace. You may read the first chapter and practice its teachings for the first week, for example, then, in the second week, add the principles of the second chapter, and so on throughout the book. Or you can read straight through the book and embark on the entire program at once. This may be your preference if you have already been living a fairly healthful life-style, or if you are eager to lose weight as quickly as is safely possible. Or, add a principle a day at a time. On the *seventh day* you will have created for yourself a new life-style, one designed to help you achieve your goal of healthier, slimmer, and happier living.

Chapter 9 is a shopping guide, including help on how to find some ingredients that may be unfamiliar to you.

Our hope is to give you a unique program and the full benefit of both Chris's twenty years of study and practice as a Seventh-Day Adventist health educator and my own perspective as a non-Seventh-Day Adventist and a "beginning student of health," who has asked many of the questions you will have, and who has had experience with putting these principles into practice.

—Jan Hoffman

THE
SEVENTH-DAY
DIET

1

· *Principle No. 1* ·

Eat a Good Breakfast

It is the custom and order of society to take a
slight breakfast. But this is not the best way to treat
the stomach. . . . Make your breakfast correspond
more nearly to the heartiest meal of the day.
—Ellen G. White

The first step in your weight- and cholesterol-management program is learning how to eat a good breakfast. *This* weight-loss program begins by *adding* a meal!

Is there really anything new to learn about eating breakfast? You may think not. But often people either skip breakfast or swallow a toast-and-coffee combination that bears little resemblance to the kind of meal that will build energy and trim fat.

The fact is, most of us "fuel up" *after* the day's work is done. This is just the opposite of what should be! A large meal early in the day will provide fuel for the body *when it is needed.* After all, breakfast means "break the fast." You've been fasting all night; now it's time to energize your body with foods that allow you to perform at peak capacity!

Performance fuel is found in the form of complex carbohydrates, plant foods such as whole grains, fresh fruits, and vegetables. Unfortunately, the average American gets only 22 percent of his or her daily calories from complex carbohydrates—a fraction of what he or she really needs. According to the Senate Select Committee on Nutrition and Human Needs, Americans need to increase their complex carbohydrate consumption by as much as 100 percent. We need to get, at the very least, half of our calories from complex carbohydrates instead of from "foodless" convenience foods. The greatest percentage of our whole carbohydrate foods should be eaten at breakfast time.

3

Between one-third and one-half of our calories should come from breakfast alone!

American consumption of complex carbohydrates has dropped dramatically since the beginning of the century. On average, Americans consume 25 percent fewer complex carbohydrates than we did in 1909. Scientists suspect that this helps explain the escalating rates of heart disease in our nation. Dr. Jeremiah Stamler of the Department of Community Health and Preventive Medicine at Northwestern University Medical School has found lower cholesterol levels in Europeans, whose diets contain a greater proportion of complex carbohydrates. Researchers William and Sonja Connor of Oregon Health Services University in Portland state that "most population groups with a low incidence of coronary heart disease consume from 65 to 85 percent of their total energy in the form of carbohydrates derived from whole grains and tubers."

Eating a hearty breakfast according to our breakfast plan will make it easy for you to enjoy a major share of those complex carbohydrates. Without this nutrient-rich fuel (most wisely eaten at the first part of the day when energy needs are highest), you may become more susceptible to some of the chronic degenerative diseases that plague the greater percentage of Americans.

One reason a high complex carbohydrate diet helps reduce the risk of a number of diseases is that it is low in sugar and fat. Also the soluble fiber in such a diet (as in oats, beans, and apples) reduces the risk of heart disease, while the insoluble fiber (as in wheat bran) reduces the risk of colon cancer.

"Eat breakfast like a king, lunch like a queen, and supper like a pauper!" say Seventh-Day Adventists. They have long been convinced that the digestive system is better equipped to manage a large quantity of food at the beginning of the day than it is at any other meal. They believe that *when we eat* is as important as *what we eat,* and that the body will function more energetically and joyfully in harmony with the natural rhythm of the digestive cycle. After a good night's sleep, the body is ready for a substantial early meal. The mind and muscles have been rested, and so has the stomach; there has been time for the digestive enzymes to be stored in concentrated supply.

One popular diet and life-style program that claims to be based on natural body cycles dictates that nothing be eaten before noon except fruit, that lunch be light, and that the heavy meal of the day be eaten in the evening. We feel this interpretation of natural body cycles is a mistake. The authors of the program have recognized that natural body cycles do exist, but they have attempted to force these cycles into a shape that has much to do with preexisting life-style patterns and little to do with real health. The plan also gives no consideration to those who have blood sugar problems (hypoglycemia or diabetes) and may become weak and even ill if food is withheld till the end of the day.

Some people who suffer from hypoglycemic symptoms will find blessed relief simply by eating a good, big breakfast. Hypoglycemia, or chronic low blood sugar, can result from several things, including when we eat *and* what we eat. Skipping breakfast and downing a cup of coffee or grabbing a piece of toast—or worse, a sweet roll—can trigger low blood sugar responses. The combination of caffeine, white flour, and sugar sends a flood of insulin into the system. Blood sugar levels instantly rise, only to drop dramatically two hours later. The normal pancreas, through its sugar-regulating hormones, is able to keep the body's blood sugar levels in balance. But when it is incessantly abused by meal skipping and snacking on undesirable foods, the pancreas literally loses its capacity to respond. At first, through exhaustion, it panics and produces too much insulin, and eventually it goes on strike. Overburdened, it becomes a defective regulator, ultimately failing to produce utilizable insulin. Thus hypoglycemia, the exact opposite of diabetes, is often the forerunner of diabetes.

Hypoglycemic symptoms may include headaches, drowsiness, crankiness, lightheadedness—even tremors and blackouts in severe cases. For some, simply eating a good breakfast will eliminate these symptoms entirely.

Even for those who are not classified as hypoglycemic, skipping breakfast often results in inefficiency, tiredness, weakness, and confusion. These can have terrible effects on one's mood and personality!

Says developmental psychologist Ernesto Pollitt of the University of California at Davis, "It seems clear that although many abilities are not affected at all, children who don't eat breakfast have difficulty with attention tasks and on solving certain kinds of problems."

The "Alameda Studies" have been embraced by Adventists as classics in the study of health. Researchers Nedra B. Belloc of the California State Department of Health and Lester Breslow of the School of Public Health at UCLA studied seven thousand Americans living in Alameda County, California, in 1965, collecting comprehensive data relating health habits and longevity. Nine years later a follow-up study was performed. Among the seven health practices examined was that of eating breakfast regularly. Though it is very difficult to isolate the effects of a single health habit, Drs. Belloc and Breslow observed that there was a decided trend toward lower mortality rates among those people who ate breakfast regularly when compared to those who said they ate breakfast "sometimes, rarely, or never."

If you are a parent, observe your own children and see how their mood and general functioning are affected by a good breakfast or the lack of one. (If they have stuffed themselves with junk food the night before, this may not be a fair study!)

Do some research on your own body for a few days. Try eating a good breakfast, and see how your work performance fares throughout the morning. Observe also your energy level and your general mood.

For many people, feeling good may be the most important result of all. How many children have been scolded for crankiness when a simple peanut butter and banana sandwich would have painlessly improved their mood? How many people who are trials to their families and friends might acquire a reputation for being mild and reasonable if they had a steaming bowl of oatmeal with fresh fruit every morning? It has become more and more clear that body chemistry can have profound effects on one's disposition.

It is said that we have wiped out malnutrition in America, and it is true that we do not see many American children with the advanced diseases of malnutrition found in many third-world countries. But many of us suffer from feelings of lassitude, low energy, nervousness, from a slight vitamin deficiency rather than a startling one—and symptoms that don't show up at all until they surface in deadly degenerative diseases. The right kind of breakfast will do much to relieve these problems.

Perhaps you have the sunniest of dispositions, are rarely tired and confused, and feel good most of the time. Perhaps the only thing that's making you irritable is that we haven't gotten around to telling you how eating breakfast will help you lose weight!

Here's how it works. First, by letting yourself get ravenous during the first half of the day, you are likely to more than make up for it during the rest of the day, often with fatty or sugary snacks. If you eat a substantial meal in the morning, chances are good that you will end up eating *fewer* total calories throughout the day. A plant-based breakfast of whole grains, fresh fruits, nuts, and seeds contains, on the average, 400 fewer calories than other meals during the day, while providing a higher portion of vitamins and minerals.

Eating a good breakfast can help minimize or eliminate problems with bingeing or compulsive eating. Fresh fruits and whole grains are high in water content and bulk, providing a greater satiety value than do foods high in fat and sugar. This means that these foods will reduce the desire for high-calorie snacks.

There are studies that show that people who skip breakfast are more likely to be obese than those who eat breakfast. One 1988 study of 339 French children showed that obese children ate less at breakfast and more at dinner than did their leaner peers.

Finally, there is evidence that calories ingested in the early part of the day will not put on as much weight as the very same calories ingested in the latter part of the day. We used to be told that a calorie is a calorie is a calorie. But there is evidence that calories may be treated differently by the body depending on the time of day they are taken in. In a study at the National Institutes of Health, two of three obese individuals who were given 400 calories at 8 A.M. lost one kilogram more weight in ten days *and more body fat* than their peers who received the same meal at 5 P.M. In another study at the University of Minnesota, six people were placed on a 2,000-calorie-a-day diet. During the first half of the experiment, the entire allotment of daily calories was eaten at breakfast; during the rest of the experiment, all the calories were taken at supper. All subjects lost weight when their meal was taken at breakfast. The *same meal,* taken in the evening, caused four of the six to *gain* weight, while two of the six lost less than they had when they had eaten breakfast. The difference was an average of 2½ pounds per week.

The beauty of this principle is that we may indulge in a filling, delicious meal without feeling guilty. It is not that we will lose weight *in spite of* eating a big breakfast—we will lose weight, at least in part, *because* of our big breakfast!

Perhaps eating breakfast seems distasteful to you. That's because you have eaten too much the night before! Try eating dinner earlier and lighter—or try skipping dinner altogether. The *last* meal of the day should be eaten at least several hours before bedtime so the stomach will be empty in the morning.

Most people have not given a lot of thought to the amount of time food stays in the digestive system. But the truth is, after a few hours of constant work, our stomachs need the opportunity to rest their muscles and restore a supply of digestive juices before the next meal. The process of digestion involves an intricate balancing act of enzymes, hormones, and muscular work. If our stomachs' delicate machinery obtains no rest, poor assimilation occurs and disease inevitably takes us hostage. The average person goes to bed in the company of lunch, late evening dinner, and snacks from all day long! Toxic by-products result, with detrimental effects on the brain and other vital organs.

If you find that you feel nauseated in the morning or have no appetite even if you haven't eaten much the night before, try using the very earliest part of the morning for something that requires mental effort or for physical exercise—with a big breakfast afterward as your reward.

Immediately upon arising, please drink a glass of water. If you want to do it the way the long-lived Seventh-Day Adventists do it, drink a glass of *warm* water—*very* warm water, perhaps with a squeeze of fresh lemon. Many drink *two* glasses of warm water before breakfast! If you're not in the habit of drinking warm water, it may seem unappetizing at first. We suggest you begin with half a glassful, then graduate to a small glass. If you can't overcome your aversion to warm water, drink a glass of cool water. Water is an essential part of this program, and it is very important that you have some when you first get up. Drinking a glass or two of warm water prepares the stomach for the digestion of breakfast. Maximum weight loss depends on food being digested and moved out of the system as rapidly as possible—and water helps by stimulating peristaltic movement of the digestive tract. Also, on a chilly morning you may be grateful for warm water and its warming effect on your body.

And now it's time for breakfast.

1 slice whole-grain bread

1 teaspoon nut butter

½ to 1 cup whole-grain cereal or other protein food

1 citrus fruit

1 other fruit

1 glass (8 ounces) milk

1 slice of whole-grain bread: Choose grains from wheat, oat, rye, millet, cornmeal, and other whole grains. A waffle may be substituted for the bread.

1 teaspoon nut butter: The nut butter may be made from peanuts, almonds, cashews, sesame seeds, or other nuts and seeds—with nothing added other than a little salt.

½ to 1 cup of whole-grain cereal or other protein food: The whole-grain cereal may be a simple grain, or mixed grains, or granola. It is best to choose a grain different from that in the bread you eat. Or instead of cereal you may eat any vegetable protein such as tofu or an extra waffle with nut butter.

1 citrus fruit: The most common citrus fruits are, of course, oranges, grapefruits, and tangerines. The whole fruit (eaten whole, cut up, or blended in a "smoothie") is preferable to the juice alone.

1 other fruit: Choose from what is available fresh and in season— apples, strawberries, pears, peaches, apricots, pineapple, blueberries, grapes, raspberries, bananas, etc. One-half to 1 cup of cut-up fruit or berries equals one serving.

1 glass of milk: Please choose from skim milk, nut milk, soy milk, cultured buttermilk, or lowfat yogurt. If you don't eat dairy products, you will, of course, choose the soy or nut milk. If you do eat dairy products, please choose from the low-fat varieties.

Most of the time you will follow the simplest version of this breakfast plan: Toast with nut butter, cereal with milk, and two fruits.

Once or twice a week you may wish to try one of the delicious recipes in this section. A single serving of any recipe from this section may substitute for either the bread or the cereal, and a double serving will substitute for both. (The servings for the waffle and French toast recipes are calculated as double servings; it is assumed you will want to replace both bread and cereal with these special dishes.)

Your family will love the savory aromas beckoning them to the breakfast table!

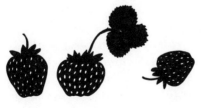

• RECIPES •

Some notes on waffles: To avoid disaster it is best to season your new waffle iron before using for the first time (this may not be necessary with Teflon-coated irons). Spray your heated waffle iron with no-stick vegetable-oil spray and continue to heat for 3 to 5 minutes. Repeat this procedure twice more before pouring the waffle batter.

Making waffles is easy once you get a feel for exactly how long your particular iron takes, and how much batter to pour for each waffle. The batter will thicken as it sits, and it may be necessary to add a little water before pouring each waffle. Keep the batter in the blender so you can give it a little whirl before pouring each new waffle.

Some people prefer waffles a little less crisp than they are right off the iron. Drape some plastic wrap over the waffles before serving, and they will soften nicely.

We have had good luck with freezing leftover waffles in food storage bags, then unwrapping them and placing them in a 350-degree oven to heat and crisp for a few minutes on each side before serving. This is a good idea for single people who love waffles in the morning but who don't want to get out the waffle iron every time the craving strikes.

Light and Heavenly Oatmeal Waffles

This is the breakfast recipe I use when I want to impress someone who is suspicious of "health food." Most whole-grain waffles are heavy and dense because they are made with whole-wheat flour and soy flour. They have been known to resemble bricks! These waffles, however, are made with rolled oats, which give a lighter result in baking. They are irresistible when spread with a little peanut butter and topped with one of the fruit syrups in Chapter 2—or make your own syrup by mixing a mashed, very ripe banana with your favorite fruit (peaches and strawberries are great) and a little juice. Or you may choose to use one of the fruit-sweetened syrups, jellies, or preserves that are on the market.

You may wonder about the use of coconut in some of these recipes. Usually it is an optional ingredient. You may have heard that it is bad for you because it is high in saturated fat. A number of studies have demonstrated that if there is no cholesterol in the diet (as in a total vegetarian diet with no animal products), the saturated fat in coconut does not elevate blood cholesterol. However, if you are eating a fair amount of animal products, it would be safer to omit the coconut.

The honey in the recipe is not for sweetening but to aid in browning. Please be sure to use ground *coriander—more on this often-used seasoning in Chapter 9.*

2 **cups rolled oats**

2 **cups water**

2 **tablespoons Soyagen (soy protein powder) or ¼ cup frozen liquid egg substitute (equivalent to 1 egg), thawed**

1 **tablespoon canola oil**

1 **teaspoon liquid lecithin**

1 **teaspoon honey**

1 **teaspoon vanilla extract**

½ **teaspoon ground coriander**

½ **teaspoon salt**

2 **tablespoons shredded unsweetened coconut (optional)**

Heat waffle iron.

Place all ingredients in blender and blend until creamy.

Brush waffle iron lightly with vegetable oil or use a no-stick vegetable-oil spray. Pour in enough batter to make one waffle (try ⅝ cup of batter for a 7-inch round waffle iron). Bake without opening for 7 to 10 minutes or until golden brown. (Be prepared to burn or undercook a waffle or two! You will learn from experience the precise baking time for your waffle iron.)

Serve with one of the fruit toppings in Chapter 2, or try a fruit-sweetened syrup, jelly, or preserves.

Makes about 4 large waffles, to serve 4

Sunday Sunflower Waffles

Here is another waffle recipe that is worth a rhapsody or two.

The millet comes in little yellow "pearls" and can be found in any health food store and many grocery stores. It adds protein and a little crunch to the waffle. The sunflower seeds provide a distinctly different flavor.

1½ cups rolled oats
2 cups water
¼ cup uncooked millet
¼ cup shelled raw
   sunflower seeds
2 tablespoons Soyagen
   (soy protein powder)
   or ¼ cup frozen
   liquid egg substitute
   (equivalent to 1 egg),
   thawed

2 tablespoons finely
   shredded
   unsweetened coconut
1 tablespoon canola oil
1 teaspoon liquid lecithin
1 teaspoon ground
   coriander
1 teaspoon vanilla extract
1 teaspoon honey
½ teaspoon salt

Heat waffle iron and coat with no-stick vegetable-oil spray.
Blend all ingredients in blender until creamy.
Pour into waffle iron and bake without opening for 7 to 10 minutes, or until golden brown.   ***Makes about 4 waffles, to serve 4***

Crunchy Almond Waffles

If you delight in the taste of almonds, this will be your favorite waffle recipe!

1½ cups rolled oats
2 cups water
¼ cup uncooked millet
¼ cup sliced almonds
2 tablespoons finely
   shredded,
   unsweetened coconut
2 tablespoons Soyagen
   (soy protein powder)
   or ¼ cup frozen
   liquid egg substitute
   (equivalent to 1 egg),
   thawed

1 tablespoon canola oil
1 teaspoon liquid lecithin
1 teaspoon honey
½ teaspoon almond
   extract
¼ teaspoon orange
   extract
½ teaspoon salt

Heat waffle iron and coat with no-stick vegetable-oil spray.

Blend all ingredients in blender until creamy.

Pour into waffle iron and bake without opening for 7 to 10 minutes, or until golden brown. *Makes about 4 waffles, to serve 4*

Cashew French Toast

This is the first of many delicious recipes that contain cashews. Raw cashews are high in protein and relatively low in fat and are the key to making creamy sauces and batters without using dairy products. Unfortunately, they are also the only nuts that need to be well rinsed, as they may be grown under conditions that are less sanitary than one would like.

To cut down on the expense of these versatile nuts, you may buy them in pieces rather than whole, in bulk at your local health food store.

You will not taste the dates in this recipe and those that follow; they are added simply for texture and sweetness. Far superior to simple sugars, they contain fiber, vitamins, and minerals as well as sweetening power. If you buy them pitted, you might want to give each one a little investigative squeeze before you put it in the blender. Your blender may handle the occasional random pit very well, but it makes a terrible racket!

The use of glass baking dishes makes it convenient to look underneath the dish to see if the French toast has browned.

2 cups water
1 cup raw cashews, well rinsed
¼ cup pitted dates
2 tablespoons frozen orange juice concentrate, thawed
1 teaspoon ground coriander

1 teaspoon vanilla extract
Pinch of salt
2 tablespoons shredded unsweetened coconut (optional)
12 slices whole-wheat bread

Preheat oven to 400°F.

Place water, cashews, dates, orange juice concentrate, coriander, vanilla, salt, and optional coconut in blender; blend until creamy. Pour into wide, shallow bowl.

Dip bread slices into cashew cream, being sure to coat them thoroughly. The batter will be thick, something like pancake batter. A gentle dipping technique is better than the dunking you may give the bread when using other, thinner French toast batters. The idea is to thinly *coat* each side of the slice of bread; use a knife to spread the batter on the bread if that makes it easier.

Place coated bread slices in lightly oiled glass baking dish or on stainless-steel cookie sheet and bake until golden brown on underside, 8 to 12 minutes. Turn slices and brown other side, 5 to 8 minutes. Some people like to complete the baking with a few seconds under the broiler for a golden brown crust. Watch closely to make sure it doesn't get *too* brown!

Serve with one of the fruit toppings given in Chapter 2, or with one of the fruit-sweetened syrups on the market.

Makes 12 pieces, to serve 6

Peanut-Date French Toast

Here's a French toast recipe for peanut-butter lovers.

1½ cups water
1 cup natural peanut butter
¼ cup pitted dates
1 teaspoon ground coriander

½ teaspoon vanilla extract
¼ teaspoon lemon extract
1 very ripe medium-size banana (optional)
12 slices whole-wheat bread

Preheat oven to 400°F.

Place water, peanut butter, dates, coriander, vanilla and lemon extracts, and optional banana in blender and blend until creamy. (Batter should be consistency of pancake batter.) Pour into wide, shallow bowl.

Dip bread into peanut cream, or spread peanut cream on both sides of bread with knife.

Place in lightly oiled glass baking dish or on stainless-steel cookie sheet and bake until golden brown on underside (8 to 12 minutes); turn and brown other side. A few seconds under the broiler will result in a golden brown crust, as described in the previous recipe.

Serve with one of the fruit toppings in Chapter 2 or with a fruit-sweetened syrup.   ***Makes 12 pieces, to serve 6***

Country-Time Bread Pudding

Here is another breakfast recipe that can double as dessert.

Depending on the size and density of the bread you use, it may take a little less than a loaf of bread to yield 6 cups of bread cubes. The easy way to make the bread cubes is to toast sliced bread in the toaster, then cut into 1-inch squares (the pieces will not be perfect cubes, of course, unless your bread is sliced 1 inch thick). Or you may cut up the bread and place on a baking sheet in a 350°F oven for 10 to 15 minutes, tossing occasionally, till lightly toasted.

6 cups whole-wheat bread
    in 1-inch cubes, lightly
    toasted
1 cup raisins
1 cup peeled, chopped
    apple

½ cup chopped pecans
¼ cup finely shredded
    unsweetened coconut
    (optional)
1 recipe Sweet Cashew
    Cream (recipe follows)

Preheat oven to 350°F.

Place the bread cubes, raisins, chopped apple, pecans, and optional coconut in large bowl. Add Sweet Cashew Cream and stir until evenly moistened. Pour into lightly oiled 13 x 9-inch baking dish.

Bake for 45 minutes.   ***Makes 8 to 10 servings***

Sweet Cashew Cream

As with other date-sweetened recipes, you may control the sweetness of this cream by using more or fewer dates. Try Sweet Cashew Cream on hot breakfast cereal.

If you like, you may add a thin strip of orange peel to the blender with the rest of the ingredients, and let the blender do the grating!

¾ cup raw cashews,
well rinsed
¾ cup hot water
2 cups cool water
¾ cup pitted dates
2 tablespoons frozen
orange juice
concentrate, thawed
1½ teaspoons vanilla
extract

1 teaspoon grated orange
peel
½ teaspoon ground
coriander
Dash almond extract
(approximately
⅛ teaspoon)

Blend cashews and hot water in blender until smooth, approximately 4 minutes.

Add cool water, dates, orange juice concentrate, and flavorings. Blend until creamy. *Makes about 4 cups*

Turn-of-the-Century Fruited Nut Gems

Gems were popular in Ellen White's day, and are still a favorite Adventist treat. They are good! The walnuts acquire a toasty flavor in the oven, and the raisins add just the right amount of sweetness.

Seventh-Day Adventists teach that baking powder or baking soda should not be used because both these leavening agents destroy important B vitamins in the baking process. Therefore, it is important to remember to mound these gems in their pans, for they will not rise any higher.

If you don't like the flavor, you may omit the banana. The gems will be just as good, though they will be much more crumbly and will require careful lifting from the pans with a spoon.

You may substitute one gem for your breakfast slice of bread.

1½ cups rolled oats
1 large apple, peeled and
grated

1 ripe banana, mashed
(optional)
½ cup raisins

<table>
<tr><td>½ cup chopped walnuts</td><td>1 teaspoon ground coriander</td></tr>
</table>

½ cup chopped walnuts
¼ cup canola oil
2 tablespoons finely shredded unsweetened coconut

1 teaspoon ground coriander
1 teaspoon grated orange peel
½ teaspoon salt

Preheat oven to 375°F.

Mix all ingredients thoroughly and let stand for 10 minutes. Spoon into lightly oiled cups of muffin tin, mounding each muffin above surface of pan; press firmly with your hand to mold.

Bake for 30 minutes, or until lightly browned.

Makes 6 to 8 gems

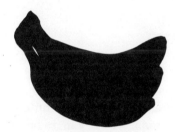

Sunrise Crunchy Granola

This special granola contains no honey or oil. It is sweetened with dried fruits and fruit juice concentrate, and combines seeds and grains for maximum protein and fiber. It is best to buy the ingredients at a good health food store, which will have all the seeds and grains in bins, ready to be scooped into bags in the desired amounts.

The recipe makes quite a large amount. It will require three good-size baking dishes if you bake it all at once. A large stockpot is perfect for mixing. Our children enjoy mixing it up with their hands. To make a smaller amount, halve the ingredients.

If you do not want to leave the granola to bake overnight, bake it at 225°F for 2 hours, or until golden and crisp. Stir occasionally to obtain uniform browning and crispness.

This granola tastes best fresh, and should be refrigerated in airtight containers. It can also be frozen in portions that are most convenient for your needs.

5 cups rolled oats
2 cups wheat flakes (or
    2 more cups rolled
    oats)
1 cup oat bran
1 cup raw sunflower seeds
½ cup raw sesame seeds
1 cup whole or sliced
    almonds
2 cups finely shredded
    unsweetened coconut
1 cup water
½ cup raw cashews, well
    rinsed

2 cups pitted dates
1 can (12 ounces) frozen
    unsweetened
    pineapple juice
    concentrate, thawed
2 teaspoons vanilla extract
1 teaspoon almond extract
1 teaspoon ground
    coriander
½ teaspoon salt
2 cups raisins

Preheat oven to 170°F.

Place first seven ingredients in very large bowl and mix thoroughly.

Make the fruit cream: Place remaining ingredients, except for raisins, in blender and blend for several minutes until creamy.

Mix blended fruit cream with dry ingredients until they are lightly and evenly moistened. (It is best to use your hands for this!)

Spread mixture in three large baking dishes about 1 inch deep.

Place the pans in the oven before bedtime. The granola will be ready at sunrise and the house will smell delicious! Toss raisins together with granola after removing from oven.

Makes 40 servings

Creamy Fruited Millet Cereal

This is a hot cereal that is a little exotic and quite tasty—for those who think they don't like hot cereal.

You may wish to serve this to a friend for breakfast with sliced grapefruit or strawberries on the side, and nut-buttered toast.

3 to 3½ cups water
½ teaspoon salt
½ teaspoon ground
    coriander
1 cup raw millet

½ cup raisins
½ cup unsweetened
    crushed pineapple,
    undrained
1 teaspoon vanilla extract

¼ cup finely shredded
   unsweetened coconut
   (optional)
Milk, soy milk, or orange
   or other fruit juice

¼ to ½ cup chopped
   pecans

Bring water to a boil, add salt and coriander, and stir in millet. Simmer, covered, over low heat for 15 minutes.

Add raisins, pineapple, vanilla, and optional coconut. Simmer, covered, for 8 to 10 minutes more. If mixture becomes too thick, stir in a little more water.

Spoon into bowls and cover with milk, soy milk, orange juice, or other fruit juice to serve. Garnish with chopped pecans.

Makes 6 servings

Early Morning Oatmeal Special

2½ cups water
½ teaspoon salt
1 cup rolled oats
½ cup raisins
1 large apple, peeled and
   shredded, or ½ cup
   unsweetened crushed
   pineapple, drained
1 ripe banana, mashed
¼ cup finely shredded
   unsweetened coconut
   (optional)

1 teaspoon vanilla extract
1 teaspoon ground
   coriander
½ teaspoon lemon extract
Milk, soy milk, or
   orange or apple juice
¼ to ½ cup chopped
   pecans

Bring water to boil, add salt, and stir in rolled oats. Cook over low heat, covered, for 15 minutes.

Stir in fruit, coconut, and flavorings. Simmer, covered, for 10 more minutes. If mixture thickens too much, it may be necessary to stir in a little more water.

Spoon into bowls and cover with milk, soy milk, orange juice, or apple juice to serve. Granish with chopped pecans.

Makes 6 servings

Millet Pineapple Crumble

This is a traditional Adventist favorite.

After measuring out a cup of cooked millet, there will be a little left over. This may be saved in the refrigerator and added to hot cereals or roasts (see page 113); or use it to make a thinner batch of the millet cream in this recipe—it's delicious on hot cereals.

1½ to 2 cups water
½ cup raw millet
1¼ cups unsweetened
    pineapple juice
¼ cup pitted dates
1 teaspoon vanilla extract
1 teaspoon ground
    coriander
¼ teaspoon lemon extract

¼ teaspoon salt
4 cups Sunrise Crunchy
    Granola or other
    granola, preferably
    fruit-sweetened
3 to 4 bananas, sliced
2 cups unsweetened
    crushed pineapple,
    drained

Bring water to boil and add millet. Simmer, covered, till cooked, about 15 minutes. If mixture thickens too quickly, it may be necessary to stir in a little more water. Measure out 1 cup cooked millet and place in blender.

To millet in blender add pineapple juice, dates, flavorings, and salt. Blend until creamy.

Lightly oil 13 x 9-inch baking dish. Spread 2 cups of the granola evenly on bottom of dish. Layer with crushed pineapple, bananas, and millet mixture. Top with remaining 2 cups granola.

Serve warmed (in 350°F oven for 12 minutes) or chilled (several hours or overnight). ***Makes 8 servings***

California Golden Fruited Toast Cups

You may come across some delicious and unusual finds in the dried fruit section of your health food store. Try them in this recipe.

8 slices whole-wheat
    bread

Nut butter (almond,
    peanut, cashew)

2 cups mixed dried fruit
(pineapples, dates,
peaches, pears,
apples, figs)
1 teaspoon vanilla extract

¼ teaspoon lemon extract
2½ cups unsweetened
pineapple juice
1 tablespoon arrowroot

Make toast cups: Preheat oven to 400°F. Trim crusts from bread and press trimmed bread slices into lightly oiled cups of muffin tin. Bake ten minutes, or until lightly toasted. Remove from oven, cool slightly, and place a teaspoonful of nut butter in each toast cup.

Make filling: Stir together dried fruit, flavorings, and 2 cups of the pineapple juice in saucepan. Simmer over low heat, stirring occasionally, until fruit softens, about 5 minutes. Combine remaining ½ cup juice with arrowroot and add slowly to fruit, stirring. Continue to stir until arrowroot is cooked and fruit mixture is thickened.

Spoon fruit filling into toast cups.

Makes 8 toast cups, to serve 4 to 8

Country-Style Breakfast Beans

This is another wonderful recipe that cooks itself at night and greets you with a delicious aroma when you wake in the morning. It makes a good breakfast served on whole-wheat toast, with fresh fruit on the side.

Leftover beans may be frozen in convenient portions and saved to serve over potatoes or rice, or used as part of an entrée.

If you prefer to cook the beans the traditional way, please see the table on page 111.

1 pound dried Great
Northern beans
¼ cup raw cashews, well
rinsed
¼ cup water
2 teaspoons salt
2 teaspoons Bakon
seasoning

1 teaspoon ground
coriander
2 teaspoons dried sweet
basil
1 teaspoon dried sage
½ teaspoon garlic powder
1 package natural onion-
soup mix (optional)

Rinse beans and pick them over. Place in crockpot.

Place cashews and water in blender and blend until creamy. Add mixture to beans along with remaining ingredients.

Cover with cold water to 2 inches above beans.

Cook in crockpot on high setting overnight (approximately 7 to 8 hours).

Serve over whole-grain toast.   *Makes 10 servings*

Breakfast Oat-Burger Sausage

This recipe does not pretend to be sausage, though it uses the same seasoning found in sausage, and satisfies the desire for something chewy and savory.

One way to form the patties is to flatten the oat mixture on waxed paper, about ⅜ inch thick, then cut with a juice glass or biscuit cutter.

This recipe makes a large amount. Extra patties can be baked and frozen, to be heated at a moment's notice. To make a smaller quantity, halve the ingredients.

4 cups water
1 cup chopped walnuts
½ cup soy sauce
¼ cup nutritional yeast
   flakes
⅓ cup canola oil
2 teaspoons Bakon
   seasoning
2 teaspoons ground
   coriander

2 teaspoons ground sage
1 tablespoon dried sweet
   basil, or 2 tablespoons
   fresh
1 teaspoon ground cumin
1 teaspoon garlic powder
½ teaspoon dried thyme
1 package natural onion-
   soup mix
4 cups rolled oats

Preheat oven to 350°F.

Place all ingredients except rolled oats in large pot and bring to slow boil.

Add rolled oats to boiling mixture and stir until thoroughly mixed. Remove immediately from heat, cover, and set aside.

When cool enough to handle, knead mixture with hands and shape into sausagelike patties.

Place in oiled baking dishes or on stainless-steel cookie sheets and bake for 15 minutes on each side.   *Makes 30 patties*

How to Cook Whole Grains

The following chart will be of use to those who want to try cooking whole grains. The secret to cooking delicious cereals is to allow enough water to swell and soften all the starch, and to cook them long enough to soften the cellulose and develop the flavor of the grain. Don't be daunted by the long cooking time some of them require; the grains can be cooked in advance and refrigerated for a few days to be reheated when needed. The method itself is simple: Bring the water to a boil, stir in the grain and salt, let simmer uncovered for 1 to 2 minutes, then turn the heat down very low, cover tightly, and cook for the specified time without uncovering.

Grain	*Water*	*Salt*	*Cooking Time*	*Yield*
½ c. hulled barley	2 c.	¼ t.	45 min.	2¼ c.
½ c. buckwheat groats	1 c.	¼ t.	15 min.	2¼ c.
1 c. millet	2 c.	½ t.	30–35 min.	4 c.
1 c. oat groats*	3 c.	¾ t.	1 hour	2½ c.
1 c. brown rice	2 c.	½ t.	45–50 min., then let stand 5 min. without uncovering	2½ c.
⅓ c. whole rye*	2½ c.	¼ t.	6 hours	2¼ c.
½ c. triticale*	1½ c.	¼ t.	1 hr.	1⅔ c.
1 c. red cereal wheat*	4 c.	½ t.	6–8 hours	2½ c.

* Soak dry grain overnight. Or, bring to a rolling boil, cover, turn off heat, and let stand 1 hour. Then proceed as directed. (In either case, it is not necessary to drain the grain—the water used to soak may also be used to cook.)

. W O R K I N G   T H E . P R O G R A M

A couple of important suggestions as you begin: One is to peek ahead to Chapter 6 and begin walking now! By the time you work your way to Chapter 6, you will be ready to put some energy into designing an effective individual exercise program for yourself. Exercise is such an important part of this program, however, that *some* daily exercise should be performed from the very beginning.

We'd also suggest that you seek out others to undertake the program with you. A group is ideal, meeting weekly to share recipes and experiences, perhaps with a scale at the meeting place so all may measure their progress, perhaps with a leader who will do a little general organizing—and who will lead the applause as all report their progress! If you can't find a group and don't want to start one yourself, try to find a partner or friend who will follow the program with you. Talk to each other daily by phone for mutual encouragement and support, perhaps meeting for walks and occasional meals. It's easier to get discouraged on your own, and it's fun and rewarding to team up with a partner.

If you can't find a partner to follow the program with you, try to enlist your family's help. Ask them to give you encouragement and support as you try to change your eating habits, even if they are not willing to follow the program as completely as you will. (Perhaps they will become more willing as time goes by!) Invite family members and friends to accompany you on your regular walks.

Weight-control classes and other life-style management programs employing the principles outlined in this book are conducted regularly at SDA hospitals, clinics, restaurants, and churches. If you are fortunate enough to live near one of these, find out when its next weight-control class will begin.

At the very back of this book you will find a couple of charts that you may begin to use now. If you have no idea what your ideal weight should be, there is a table of desirable weights according to frame and age that can be your guide. Remember that your ideal weight will also depend on factors other than your frame and age, such as the proportion of muscle mass to fat in your body and, perhaps most importantly, the weight at which you *feel* your best! The other chart is a weight-loss record that will allow you to see your weight falling as you weigh yourself each week. Record your weight now, before you begin the program, and record it every week until you reach your goal. Also—find out what your cholesterol level is and have your blood pressure taken. Monitor your blood pressure frequently if it tends to be on the high side, and eight weeks from now, have another cholesterol reading. It is encouraging to watch these numbers fall.

· · ·

How in the world are you going to fit a big breakfast into your busy schedule? Some people get everything ready the night before and get up a little earlier than usual to allow themselves time to eat. If you exercise in the morning, please eat breakfast *after* you exercise! One executive we know, who has a treadmill and free weights in a room off his office and works out heavily before his day begins, keeps granola, bread, and peanut butter at the office and brings in milk and fruit so he can breakfast at his desk after his workout. We know many people who get up early three or four times a week and walk two or three miles before coming back home for breakfast. Some people find it most efficient to eat dinner at breakfast time. (More on this unusual idea later!)

A good granola or other whole-grain cold cereal is probably the easiest quick breakfast. If you would rather have cooked cereal, we suggest the whole-grain varieties, such as Irish oatmeal with its wonderful chewy texture, wheat flakes, or delicious millet with its high-quality protein. Of course the cooking time required for these nutritious whole grains can be a problem. Some people have solved the problem by buying small crockpots made especially for cooking one to four servings of cereal overnight. You simply put the desired amount of cereal in the pot the night before, along with the appropriate amount of water and salt, and let it cook on the lowest setting overnight. You may also add dried fruits and seasonings to the pot for flavor—raisins cooked overnight in a slow cooker become plump and almost melting in their sweetness. Top with fresh strawberries, bananas, or peaches!

Making preparations the night before will make breakfast time go more smoothly. Ingredients, for example, can be assembled and measured before bed, and the overnight cooking recommended for some of the recipes in this chapter offer not only convenience but the pleasure of waking to heavenly smells throughout the house.

You can also make breakfast more fun with a blender. As you've seen, many of the recipes in this chapter call for the use of a blender, and in Chapter 2 you will find ideas for delicious drinks and smoothies made with fruits and juices.

This may be the place to discuss the relative merits of blenders and food processors. Each type of machine can do a few things that the other cannot, but for healthful cooking with whole ingredients, we recommend the blender. When making sauces out of whole ingredients, the blender achieves a smoothness that the processor cannot duplicate. It is superior for making the fruit drinks and desserts that will satisfy your desire for sweets, and for making delicious substitutes for cheese and gravy. And its emulsifying action is essential for making a flaky whole-wheat pie crust.

On the other hand, a processor does a better job of crumbling and chopping, and its shredding and slicing disks save time when preparing vegetables for salads and casseroles.

Do you have room in your budget for both?

Here are a few simple ideas to make breakfast more appealing and delicious:

• Serve different combinations of fruit juices, such as apricot nectar with grapefruit juice, orange juice with apple juice, pineapple juice with pear nectar. Or serve pieces of fruit in a fruit juice, such as sliced bananas and grapes in orange juice, or bananas and orange slices in pineapple juice. Cut up and combine your own favorite fruits to make special fruit salads.

• You may sprinkle chopped nuts over grated raw apple, or top fresh apple slices with peanut butter (this is a favorite with children).

• A little bit of toasted wheat germ sprinkled on cooked cereal adds a nutty taste. Dates, raisins, apples, bananas, pecans, and many other fruits and nuts are delicious in hot cereal. Try unsweetened frozen fruits when fresh fruits are not available.

• SUMMARY •

1. After fasting all night, you need to energize your body with foods that will enable you to perform at peak capacity.

2. There is very strong evidence that a diet high in complex carbohydrates helps to protect against heart disease and other degenerative diseases. A good breakfast provides an ideal opportunity to take in a large share of these complex carbohydrates.

3. For many people, a good breakfast will eliminate or minimize hypoglycemic symptoms.

4. Eating a good breakfast regularly has been linked with improved work performance, elevation of mood, improvement in certain kinds of problem solving—even increased longevity.

5. Calories taken in at breakfast time are burned during the day. Weight control is more difficult when breakfast is not eaten.

6. Skipping breakfast often leads to overeating at the next meal, as well as more snacking. As a result the total calories ingested for the day may increase.

7. Food digests better early in the day, when you are most active.

• This Week's Guide to Success •

Enlist support.

Ask a friend to follow the program with you. Call each other often to give mutual encouragement and support. If you can't get a friend to join you, enlist the support of family and friends. Find out if there's an SDA weight-control class near you.

Begin to exercise.

Look ahead to Chapter 6 and begin a walking program. An exercise program usually changes as time goes by—but it's important to be *always exercising*.

Eat a good breakfast.

Breakfast should contain one-third to one-half of the day's total calories. Remember to drink a glass or two of water before breakfast.

Program your mind for success.

Pay attention to how you feel when you begin to follow the simple measures in this chapter. Take notice of your increased energy day by day as you begin meeting your body's needs.

2

· *Principle No. 2* ·

Cut Out Empty and Refined Calories

*For use in breadmaking, the superfine white
flour is not the best. Its use is neither healthful
nor economical. Fine-flour bread is lacking in
nutritive elements to be found in bread made
from the whole wheat.*
—Ellen G. White

Your lifelong battle with the bathroom scale may tip in your favor by practicing a principle that Seventh-Day Adventists have practiced for decades. It may not be the quantity of food you eat that produces those unwanted pounds, but rather the *quality*. Principle No. 2—cut out empty and refined calories—may help you to end that yo-yo experience and throw away the scale!

One of the greatest nutritional travesties of our age involves the transformation of whole natural foods into man-made products— "foodless" convenience foods. Refining and processing extends the shelf life of the product while destroying the life of the food. The end result of man's tampering with the natural structure is a product concentrated in calories but offering very little in the way of nutrition. We have seen an endless rise in the development of chronic degenerative diseases, including the greatest of all Westernized diseases: obesity. (Obesity can be called the most common "disease," and is often the foundation for serious ailments such as heart disease and diabetes, and a contributing factor in many others.) Because of our modern refining processes, food loses most of its nutritional value as it travels from the garden to the stomach and picks up a lot of undesirable baggage in the process, namely calories—*big fat empty ones!*

The biggest problem with this nutritional travesty is the loss of vitamins, minerals, and fiber. How serious is this problem? It's serious enough for us to take a look at the quality of the calories you consume on a daily basis. Just for now let's assume that your diet is equivalent to the average American's diet.

Table 1   •   *Nutrient Contributions of Foods to U.S. Diet*

Food	% of Calories	Calories/ Day	Lbs/Person/ Yr.	Tsp./Day
Sugar, syrups	12–17	525	128	33
Visible fats (oils), shortening, butter, oleo, etc.	18	550	33	
Alcohol	3	100	11	
Subtotal empty calories	38	1175	162	
Refined breads, cereals*	18–20	650		
Total empty and refined calories	58+	1825		

* Over 90% of consumption refined

If you look at Table 1, you can see that sugar and syrup amount to 12 to 17 percent of the calories consumed per day. Moving across the line, you can see that this adds up to as much as a whopping 525 calories per day, or 128 pounds of sugar per person per year.

This simply means your daily menu includes about 33 teaspoons of sugar—almost ¾ cup! You might not think that you eat that much sugar, but there's more sugar hidden in foods than you may realize. Do you put ketchup on your french fries, burgers, beans, and everything? Then you may be pouring as much as 65 percent sugar on your food. What about your kids' favorite cereal? Your little darlings may be eating candy for breakfast—many brands are 40 to 68 percent sugar. Have a dish of canned corn or canned soup for lunch? Sprinkle your salad with bottled salad dressing? There's sugar in it. Sugar comes disguised in modern food in every imaginable way. As a general rule of thumb, all refined, processed convenience foods contain sugar.

Table 2 • *Some Hidden Sources of Sugar* *

Food	Size Portion	Teaspoons Sugar
Cola drinks	1 (6-oz. bottle)	3½
Ginger ale	1 (6-oz. bottle)	5
Orangeade	1 (8-oz. glass)	5
Soda pop	1 (8-oz. glass)	5
Angel food cake	1 piece (4 oz.)	7
Banana cake	1 piece (2 oz.)	2
Chocolate cake, plain	1 piece (4 oz.)	6
Chocolate cake, iced	1 piece (4 oz.)	10
Coffee cake	1 piece (4 oz.)	4½
Cupcake, iced	1 cupcake	6
Fruit or pound cake	1 piece (4 oz.)	5
Jelly roll	1 piece (2 oz.)	2½
Sponge cake	1 piece (1 oz.)	2
Strawberry shortcake	1 serving	4
Brownies, unfrosted	1 (¾ oz.)	3
Chocolate cookies	1 cookie	1½
Fig Newtons	1 cookie	5
Gingersnaps	1 cookie	3
Macaroons	1 cookie	6
Nut cookies	1 cookie	1½
Oatmeal cookies	1 cookie	2
Chocolate eclair	1 eclair	7
Cream puff	1 cream puff	2
Doughnut, plain	1 doughnut	3
Doughnut, glazed	1 doughnut	6
Chocolate milk bar	1 (1½ oz. Hershey)	2½
Chewing gum	1 stick	½
Chocolate cream	1 piece	2
Butterscotch chew	1 piece	1
Fudge	1-oz. square	4½
Gumdrop	1 piece	2

* American Foundation for Medical-Dental Science, Los Angeles, California

Food	Size Portion	Teaspoons Sugar
Hard candy	1 oz. (5 pieces)	5
Peanut brittle	1 piece	3½
Canned apricots	4 halves & 1 T. syrup	3½
Canned fruit juices, sweetened	½ cup	2
Canned peaches	2 halves & 1 T. syrup	3½
Stewed fruits	½ cup	2
Ice cream	¼ pt. (3½ oz.)	3½
Ice cream bar	1 bar	1–7
Ice cream cone	1 cone	3½
Ice cream sundae	1 sundae	7
Malted milkshake	1 (10-oz. glass)	5
Apple butter	1 T.	1
Jelly or marmalade	1 T.	4–6
Strawberry jam	1 T.	4

The calories in all that hidden sugar can add up fast. For example, a slice of bread is only 60 calories; however, add to its ingredients refined sugar and oil, producing a cookie, and you double the calories. Refine with a little more sugar and oil and you can produce plain cake without icing for 200 calories or with icing for 370 calories. Now add more sugar, oil, and chocolate, and we have a masterpiece of refined sugar-laced calories—chocolate cake with chocolate icing, 445 calories. Topped with a counterfeit chemical version of yesteryear's ice cream, you now have 575 fat-producing calories!

Refined sugar is one of the most dangerous food items in this country and should be kept like other dangerous weapons under lock and key! It plays havoc with your nerves because it lacks the very B vitamins and minerals that are necessary for its assimilation. America's enormous appetite for sugar is also related to the increased incidence of obesity, dental caries, diabetes, depressed immune response, hypoglycemia, and an increase in triglyceride and cholesterol levels. We are serious when we suggest that life for everyone would be dramatically improved if we threw away this empty-calorie clinker.

Now let's take a look at visible fats. Keep in mind the word "visible." Most fats are hidden in cholesterol-laden cheeses, whole milk, and marbleized meats. But as the table shows, a fattening 18 percent of our calories come from *visible* fats. These include animal or vegetable shortening, butter, margarine, cooking oils, salad dressings, and mayonnaise. Moving across the line again, we can see that all this adds up to an additional 550 empty calories per day. If you cut back 500 calories a day you may be able to lose 50 pounds of extra weight in one year. Just by employing Principle No. 2 through the elimination of white sugar and visible fats alone, you can, if you need to, lose 100 pounds in one year! This is not by counting calories but by cutting out empty ones!

Over 20 percent of your calories comes from hidden fat. This means that a total of 40 percent of the calories in the average American diet —almost *half*—comes from fat. Sometimes we tell ourselves a little pat of butter or just a smidgen of mayonnaise can't have *too* many calories. The truth is, a meal can easily be doubled calorically by a little pat here and a little smidgen there of fat, as we see in Table 3.

Table 3 • *The Effect of Visible Fats*

Lettuce-and- tomato salad	20 calories	+ Mayonnaise, 1 T.	(100)	= 120 calories
Bread, 1 slice	60 calories	+ Butter, .6 T.	(60)	= 120 calories
Peas, ⅔ cup	100 calories	+ Butter, .6 T.	(60)	= 160 calories
Entrée	150 calories	+ Gravy	(100)	= 250 calories
Baked potato, 1 med.	<u>100</u> calories	+ Butter, .6 T.	(60)	= <u>160</u> calories
	430 calories	versus		810 calories

Table 1 shows another empty calorie offender—alcohol. Alcohol adds up to another 3 percent of the calories in the average diet. *Big hard empty ones!* Adding the 17 percent sugar to the 18 percent visible fat, then 3 percent alcohol, gives us a bulging 38 percent of our calories consumed as empty calories. That means that, nutritionally, 38 percent of the average American's daily diet adds up to zero!

Let's look at Table 1 again. The last item in the column is refined breads and cereals. As we examine our nutritional losses, there is none as devastating as what Adventists call the "Great Grain Robbery." Imagine that a pickpocket relieves a friend of twenty dollars and then, in a sudden impulse of generosity, gives *four* dollars back to him. Would he feel enriched or robbed? Well, this is similar to what happens during the strange metamorphosis of whole-grain wheat berries into virtually valueless white flour. As the food processing continues, loaves of fluffy white bread are manufactured to our (programmed) taste. The classic advertising term used to market those concentrated globs of white starch is "enriched." Well, let's see if our friend has been enriched or robbed as we look at Table 4.

Table 4 • *Nutrients Lost in the Refining Process of Whole Wheat*

	% Loss *		% Loss *
Vitamin B$_1$ (thiamine)	86	Folic acid	70
		Pantothenic acid	54
Vitamin B$_2$ (riboflavin)	70	Biotin	90
		Calcium	50
Niacin	86	Phosphorus	78
Iron	84	Copper	75
Vitamin B$_6$ (pyridoxine)	60	Magnesium	72
		Manganese	71

* Only vitamins B$_1$, B$_2$, niacin, and the mineral iron are added back in the enrichment process. Calculated from "Lesser Known Vitamins in Foods," *J Am Diet Assn* 38: 240–243, 1961, as compiled by Mervyn G. Hardinge and Hulda Crooks.

Table 5 makes it even clearer. Look how many more slices of enriched bread it takes to get the same amount of nutritional value found in one slice of whole-wheat bread.

Table 5

Pantothenic acid in 1 slice whole-wheat bread	=	2 slices white bread
Vitamin B$_6$	=	3
Folic acid	=	3
Magnesium	=	3.6
Copper	=	4
Phosphorus	=	5
Biotin	=	10
Vitamin E	=	20

This process cannot be accepted as enrichment when our whole grains have been depleted nutritionally this way. From the fragmentation process, we end up with less than what we had before the transformation occurred. When the food is fragmented, it is usually its fiber and nutritious components that are removed, making the remaining nutritionally inferior ingredients more concentrated. This adds more refined calories but very little nutrition.

How does this happen? The food processors take golden wheat berries and strip them of most of their vitamins, and minerals, and all of their fiber. This is done by removing the heart of the wheat kernel (the germ), an important source of B complex vitamins, vitamin E, and protein. They also remove the covering (the bran), an important source of fiber in our diet.

What's left? The endosperm, which is raw starch. Into the raw starch are infused three little synthetic chemicals—niacin, thiamine, and riboflavin—plus iron. Remember our friend in the story who was robbed of his twenty dollars, then was "enriched" by the return of four dollars?

What about the other sixteen bucks?

We can see some of these nutrient losses in Table 4, but the picture is incomplete, for other nutritional factors remain unknown. This means that the problem is probably more serious than we know. The processors have destroyed the synergy of the structure, and we don't know what we've lost! Yet people have been propagandized into believing that a popular brand of white bread "builds strong healthy bodies in twelve different ways."

We have observed the damage that the refining process does to wheat. The same robbery occurs with other grains. Some brands of store-bought cornmeal are labeled "degerminated." To the customer, that might sound as if the cornmeal has been "debugged." But "degerminated" means that the germ, the heart of the grain, has been removed to improve the keeping quality of the product. Yes, it keeps the bugs out—they won't eat something that doesn't sustain life. They're choosy little critters!

Natural whole-grain brown rice is refined into white rice through a polishing process until most of the vitamins and minerals are polished away. Consumers purchasing this flimflam version of a grain that is "ready to be served" three minutes after opening the package might do as well to eat the box—it's got just about as much nutrition in it! Even the "longer-cooking" white rice is nutritionally impoverished. The same goes for instant oats, as opposed to old-fashioned rolled oats.

Let's add up all these empty calories in the typical American diet. We'll add refined breads and cereals to the column of empty calories since the vitamins, minerals, and fiber have been stripped away, leaving our grains in nearly the same shape as our empty-calorie foods. This means that the daily empty and refined calories the average American eats totals 58 percent of the entire diet. Almost 60 percent of what you eat has virtually no nutrition! As you can plainly see, that adds up to an unnecessary 1,825 calories daily, which end up as fat on your body.

Look at Table 6. Notice that milk and milk products provide 11 percent of our total daily calories, meat provides 20 percent, and eggs another 2 percent. But milk has no fiber. Eggs have no fiber. Meat has no fiber. You see, the foods that provide the greatest percentage of vitamins, minerals, and fiber, the very foods that make a person healthy and slim, make up the smallest percentage of our daily diet.

Table 6 • U.S. Food Group Consumption

Food Group	% of Total Calories
Milk group	11
Meat	20
Eggs	2
Bread and Cereal group	20
Fruit and Vegetable group	9
Fats and oils, visible*	18
Sugar and sweeteners	12–17
Alcohol	3–5

* 18 from visible but U.S. diet is 30–37% from fat because of hidden fat in meat, milk, etc.

The solution to the fat problem is clear. A variety of whole natural vegetables, fruits, grains, beans, and nuts will help you to lose excessive weight or maintain ideal body weight!

As you begin your weight-loss program, you may find that it's hard to curb your sweet tooth all the time. In fact, even when you've made the entire program a part of your life, there will be occasions—holidays and family gatherings, for example—that call for something special. Instead of reaching for a package of cookies or a sugary cake, try one of the healthy sweets from the selection that follows.

· RECIPES ·

Please exercise some caution with the desserts in this section. Pies and cobblers should be occasional treats.

Toward the end of this section are beverages made of herb tea, juices, and fruit. These too should be limited if your goal is to lose weight rapidly, but they are infinitely more healthful than soft drinks—and infinitely more flavorful as well. They are wonderful to serve when you have company, or to replace the harmful soft drinks so many of us are addicted to.

Hidden away at the very end of this recipe section are some rich, fudgy concoctions that should be used very sparingly, and probably not at all by those who are eager to lose weight. None of them contain a gram of cholesterol—but they are very concentrated and sweet.

In fact, *most of the time* when you want to make a special sweet treat, it would be best to turn to Chapter 3 and prepare one of the simple fruit desserts in the recipe section. The more elaborate recipes in this chapter are meant for *very* special occasions—and to show your children and your guests that a delectable sweet dessert need not be laced with sugar or other refined foods.

Summer Fresh Fruit Pie

Many people are going to ask you for this recipe! It is a wonderful dish to serve guests for brunch in summer, and is one of Chris's most popular desserts.

For the best pie, choose the best fruit—ripe, flavorful, and deep in color. In wintertime when fresh fruit is not as plentiful, you may make the pie with bananas, pineapple, and frozen strawberries and peaches. Whether you are using fresh or frozen fruit, be sure to use bananas for the layer next to the crust so the juice from the other fruit won't soak into the crust.

2 cups Sunrise Crunchy
   Granola (page 17) or
   other granola,
            preferably fruit-
            sweetened

¼ cup nut butter (peanut, cashew, or almond)	1 cup sliced peaches
2 medium-size ripe bananas, sliced	1 cup blueberries
	Pineapple-Lemon Sauce (recipe follows)
1 cup sliced strawberries	¼ cup chopped pecans

Make pie crust: Preheat oven to 350°F. Make granola into crumbs by blending in blender or food processor and place in mixing bowl. Soften nut butter by heating it gently, add to granola crumbs, and mix thoroughly until crumbs are moistened. Press crumb–nut butter mixture into 9-inch pie plate and bake for 10 minutes. Remove from oven and let cool.

Layer fruit into pie crust, beginning with bananas.

Top with Pineapple-Lemon Sauce and garnish with chopped pecans.

Chill for an hour or two before serving. (You may chill it longer, but be aware that it tends to get soggy if chilled for more than a few hours.)   ***Makes one 9-inch pie, to serve 8***

Note: To save a little time you may choose not to make the granola into crumbs. Simply mix the whole granola with the softened nut butter and press it into the pan. A graham-cracker crust will also work in this recipe.

You may also shave a few minutes off preparation time by substituting a topping of thickened crushed pineapple for the Pineapple-Lemon Sauce: Pour off a little of the juice from a 20-ounce can of unsweetened crushed pineapple and mix it well with 2 tablespoons arrowroot or cornstarch. Place this mixture in a saucepan with the rest of the pineapple and juice. Bring to a slow boil, then simmer over low heat, stirring constantly, until thickened and clear, approximately 5 to 10 minutes.

Pineapple-Lemon Sauce

This sauce—warm, cool, or chilled—is also delicious over pancakes, waffles, fruitcake, cereals, or fruit.

1 cup unsweetened
    pineapple juice
2 tablespoons arrowroot
¼ teaspoon lemon extract
⅛ teaspoon salt
2 cups unsweetened
    crushed pineapple,
    undrained

3 tablespoons honey
1 tablespoon fresh lemon
    juice
1 teaspoon grated lemon
    peel

Place pineapple juice, arrowroot (or cornstarch), lemon extract, and salt in blender and blend until smooth. Pour blended mixture into 1-quart saucepan. Bring to slow boil and simmer over low heat, stirring constantly, until thickened and *clear,* approximately 5 to 10 minutes.

Remove from heat and add remaining ingredients. Mix well and cool. ***Makes approximately 3 cups***

Blueberry Syrup

This is everybody's favorite syrup, sweet and delicious. Serve over waffles, pancakes, or French toast.

When using arrowroot, it is important to cook the sauce long enough so that it not only thickens, but becomes clear; otherwise it will retain an undesirable powdery taste. Of course, the sauce will not become as clear as glass, especially if it contains other ingredients such as blueberries, but you will notice a change in appearance—a glossiness—soon after it thickens. This is the point after which you may add the other ingredients.

3½ cups fresh or
    unsweetened frozen
    blueberries
1 can (6 ounces) frozen
    apple juice
    concentrate, thawed

½ cup pitted dates
1 tablespoon arrowroot
⅛ teaspoon salt
1 teaspoon fresh lemon
    juice

If using fresh blueberries, wash them and remove stems. Set aside.

Place in blender apple juice concentrate, ½ cup of the blueberries, pitted dates, arrowroot, and salt. Blend until smooth.

Place blended mixture in saucepan and simmer over low heat, stirring constantly, until thickened and clear, approximately 5 to 10 minutes. Add rest of blueberries and lemon juice. Simmer over low heat briefly until heated (do not boil).

Makes approximately 4 cups

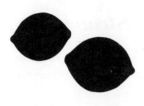

Piña Colada Fruit Cream

For a smaller amount of this delicious cream, you can halve the recipe. But before you do, you should know that we have known guests and children to drink it straight!

The lemon juice is folded in at the last so that it will help thicken the cream; blended in too quickly or too soon, it will cause the mixture to thin.

Soyagen, a soy protein powder, can be found at an Adventist Book and Nutrition Center or at a health food store. If you have trouble finding it, you may use another brand of soy protein powder or ½ cup of cashew milk or soy milk, although the cream will not be as thick.

The bananas need to be very ripe, to the point of having brown spots on the skin, so that they will be very sweet.

2 cups fresh or unsweetened canned pineapple chunks, drained if canned	¼ cup honey
	1 teaspoon ground coriander
4 medium-size very ripe bananas	1½ teaspoons vanilla extract
1 cup unsweetened pineapple juice	1½ teaspoons coconut extract
½ cup Soyagen (soy protein powder)	⅛ teaspoon salt
	1 teaspoon fresh lemon juice

Place all ingredients except lemon juice in blender and blend until very creamy.

Stop blender and slowly fold in lemon juice, stirring just a few times.

Chill. Serve over fruit salad or other dessert.

Makes approximately 4 cups

Pineapple-Strawberry Fruit Sauce

Serve as a topping for waffles, pancakes, or French toast. The sauce may be served at room temperature or slightly warmed.

3 medium-size very ripe
   bananas
1 can (20 ounces)
   unsweetened crushed
   pineapple, undrained
½ cup sliced strawberries

3 tablespoons finely
   shredded unsweetened
   coconut
1 teaspoon ground
   coriander

Mash bananas with fork until smooth. Add crushed pineapple, strawberries, coconut, and coriander. Mix thoroughly.

Makes approximately 3½ to 4 cups

Tangy Sweet Lemon Sauce

Drizzle this flavorful sauce lightly over fresh fruit, cakes, or hot cereals. The tartness of the sauce makes it especially good on very sweet foods such as Orange Date-Nut Cake (page 54).

1 cup unsweetened
   pineapple juice
2 tablespoons arrowroot
1 teaspoon grated lemon
   peel
¼ teaspoon lemon extract

½ teaspoon ground
   coriander
⅛ teaspoon salt
3 tablespoons honey
1 tablespoon fresh lemon
   juice

Place in blender pineapple juice, arrowroot, lemon peel, lemon extract, coriander, and salt. Blend thoroughly.

Place blended mixture in small saucepan. Bring to slow boil and simmer over low heat, stirring constantly, until thickened and clear.

Remove from heat and add honey and lemon juice, stirring thoroughly.　　　　　　　　　　　　***Makes approximately 1 cup***

Orange-Pineapple Sauce

1 cup orange juice, fresh if possible
2 tablespoons arrowroot
¼ teaspoon orange extract (optional)
1 teaspoon grated orange peel
⅛ teaspoon salt

2 cups unsweetened crushed pineapple, undrained
3 tablespoons honey
1 tablespoon frozen orange juice concentrate, thawed

Place in blender orange juice, arrowroot, optional extract, orange peel, and salt, and blend until smooth. Place blended mixture in 1-quart saucepan, bring to slow boil, and simmer over low heat, stirring constantly, until thickened and clear.

Remove from heat and add crushed pineapple, honey, and orange juice concentrate. Mix well and chill.

Makes approximately 3 cups

Dutch Apple-Raisin Sauce

Serve over waffles, pancakes, French toast, or hot cereal.

4 medium-size golden delicious apples
1 cup raisins
¼ cup chopped walnuts
½ cup water
¼ teaspoon vanilla extract

½ cup frozen unsweetened apple juice concentrate, thawed
½ teaspoon ground coriander

Pare, core, and thinly slice apples. Place apples, raisins, nuts, and water in 2-quart saucepan. Bring to slow boil and simmer, uncovered, over low heat for 3 to 5 minutes, stirring occasionally.

Add vanilla, apple juice concentrate, and coriander. Simmer, uncovered, for 3 minutes more, stirring occasionally. The apples should retain their shape yet turn soft and juicy.

Makes approximately 4 cups

Pineapple-Orange Sherbet

Never throw out overripe bananas! Wrap them in plastic and store them in the freezer, ready to take out and slice into the blender to make smoothies, sherbets, and other frozen desserts. If your freezer has made the bananas rock hard, it may be necessary to let them sit for a few minutes until they are of a more manageable (blendable) consistency.

Here's a sweet, flavorful sherbet that contains no trace of sugar. For a treat, garnish with nuts and fresh strawberry slices.

½ cup unsweetened apple juice

¼ cup frozen pineapple juice concentrate, thawed

3 medium-size very ripe bananas, frozen

½ cup fresh or unsweetened frozen pineapple chunks, drained if canned, frozen

Place all ingredients in blender and blend until smooth. If mixture stalls blender, it may be necessary to turn off motor and stir fruit or add just a little more juice, then continue blending. Serve immediately.

Makes 4 servings

Winter Fresh Fruit Cream

A beautiful dessert, red against green; a garnish of sliced almonds in addition to the frozen strawberries makes it look even more festive.

3 medium-size very ripe
   bananas, frozen
1 soft-ripe pear, peeled
   and cored
1 ripe avocado, pitted and
   peeled
2 tablespoons honey

½ cup unsweetened
   pineapple juice
½ teaspoon ground
   coriander
Unsweetened frozen
   sliced strawberries

Place all ingredients except strawberries in blender and blend until smooth. Serve immediately, in sherbet glasses, garnished with sliced frozen strawberries.   ***Makes 5 servings***

Iced Brazilian Banana Boats

Children love a frozen dessert with a "chocolaty" coating. The coating on this dessert is carob, much better for the children than chocolate.

Very ripe bananas
Carob Sauce (recipe
   follows)

Finely chopped nuts (try
   pecans or peanuts)

Remove skins from bananas. Wrap bananas individually in plastic wrap and place in freezer.

Unwrap frozen bananas, dip in Carob Sauce, and roll in finely chopped nuts.

Return to freezer until serving time.

Carob Sauce

This sauce is also good on waffles, peanut-butter toast, and frozen fresh fruit.

  1 cup pitted dates
2½ cups boiling water
  ½ cup roasted carob
     powder
  ¼ cup honey

1 teaspoon ground
   coriander
1 teaspoon vanilla extract
⅛ teaspoon salt

Place dates in blender; pour 1 cup of the hot water over them and leave to soften while you assemble other ingredients.

Add remaining ingredients to blender. Place lid on blender, with center insert removed. Turn on blender and immediately begin pouring in remaining 1½ cups hot water in thin stream. After all water has been added, continue to blend mixture until creamy.

Makes about 3½ cups

Flaky Pie Crust

You are about to become acquainted with the famous Flaky Pie Crust. It is excellent for both sweet and savory dishes, and it is very easy to make, compared to most other pie crust recipes. At least half the flour in it is whole wheat, and it contains no hydrogenated shortening; the shortening is made by emulsifying oil and water in the blender. Please use a blender if you have one—sometimes a food processor will emulsify the oil and water, but most of the time it won't!

This recipe makes enough for a double crust for an 8- or 9-inch pie, or a large top crust for a cobbler in a 13 x 9-inch baking dish. If you only need a single crust for a round pie, it is best to make the whole recipe and save the leftover dough in the refrigerator to be used in a day or two. We have even had good luck freezing the dough, to be thawed and rolled out when needed. Or roll out the extra dough, fill a pie plate, cover with plastic wrap, and freeze, to be baked at your convenience.

1 cup whole-wheat pastry flour	½ teaspoon salt
	½ cup water
¾ to 1 cup unbleached flour	⅓ cup vegetable oil
	1½ teaspoons lecithin

Place flours and salt in bowl and mix well.

Measure water and pour it into blender, then measure oil into measuring cup. Dip a teaspoon measure into oil and measure the lecithin with oil-coated spoon. Lecithin should slide easily off spoon into water in blender. Finally, pour oil into blender. Blend until thick and creamy (mixture should take on thickness and appearance of a glossy mayonnaise).

Add blended mixture to flours in bowl and mix with a fork. Dough should be pliable and *very moist,* but not sticky. (It is most important to have a moist, soft dough, so begin with 1¾ cups flour and add more if the dough is too sticky. If dough is right consistency to begin with, it won't be necessary to add extra flour when rolling it out.)

Spread some plastic wrap on dampened kitchen counter, enough to provide a large enough area to roll pie dough out. (It will probably be necessary to use two overlapping strips of plastic wrap.) Form dough into ball. Pat it out with your hands on the plastic wrap until you have a large, flat round, then continue with a rolling pin until dough is very thin and several inches larger than pie plate. (We've gotten so adept at handling the dough that we don't even use a rolling pin. We just pat the dough out on the plastic wrap, then cover it with a second layer of plastic wrap, continuing to pat it out firmly with the hands on the top layer of plastic wrap until the dough is very thin.)

Place your pie plate or baking dish next to rolled-out dough. Lift dough carefully by edges of plastic wrap and turn gently and smoothly into plate. Carefully peel away plastic wrap.

Makes enough pastry for a double-crust round pie,
or a single covering pastry for a 13 x 9-inch cobbler

Note: If you don't want to use unbleached flour, try oat flour or barley flour for a purist's whole-grain crust. But in any case, be sure to use whole-wheat *pastry* flour for the whole-wheat portion of the flour.

Crunchy Granola Pie Crust

An easy-to-make pie crust that you can make even easier if you leave the granola whole.

2 cups Sunrise Crunchy Granola (page 17) or other granola, preferably fruit-sweetened

2 tablespoons finely shredded unsweetened coconut (optional)

¼ cup nut butter (almond, peanut, cashew)

Preheat oven to 350°F.

Place granola in blender or food processor and process into crumbs. Transfer to large bowl and stir in optional coconut.

Warm nut butter in small saucepan over very low heat until softened. Add softened nut butter to granola crumbs and work until evenly blended. It may be necessary to use your hands for this process.

Press mixture into pie plate and bake for 10 to 12 minutes. Cool before filling. *Makes a single 9-inch crust*

Aromatic Oat-Almond Pie Crust

Here's a special fragrant pie crust that is best offset by a simple fruit filling. Try filling it with sliced fresh fruit and covering with one of the fruit sauces in this chapter.

If you don't care to grind your own almonds in the blender or food processor, you will find almond meal and almond butter at any health food store.

⅓ cup rolled oats	⅓ cup almond butter
⅓ cup whole-wheat pastry flour	2 tablespoons water
3 tablespoons flat almond slices	½ teaspoon almond extract
	¼ teaspoon vanilla extract
	⅛ teaspoon salt

Preheat oven to 350°F.

Blend rolled oats in blender until finely ground. Place ground oats in large bowl with flour and almond slices and mix thoroughly.

Add almond butter to dry ingredients and cut in with knives, pastry cutter, or fingers until blended thoroughly. Add water and extracts and blend lightly with a fork.

Press mixture evenly into 9-inch pie plate. Bake for 12 to 15 minutes. *Makes a single 9-inch crust*

Deep-Dish Blueberry Pie

This is the easiest of our fruit pies, because blueberries don't need as much preparation as do apples and peaches. If fresh blueberries are unavailable, you may substitute frozen blueberries.

The amounts given here will make a 13 x 9-inch deep-dish

pie, with a recipe of Flaky Pie Crust for a single covering crust. Halve the filling amounts to make a deep double-crust 9-inch round pie or a deep-dish pie in an 8-inch square pan with a single covering crust (in which case, halve the Flaky Pie Crust recipe too).

10¼ cups fresh or frozen
    unsweetened
    blueberries
1 can (12 ounces) frozen
    apple juice
    concentrate, thawed
1 cup pitted dates
¼ cup arrowroot

1 teaspoon ground
    coriander
1 teaspoon vanilla
    extract
½ teaspoon salt
1 recipe Flaky Pie Crust
    (page 44)

Preheat oven to 350°F.

If using fresh blueberries, rinse, drain, and set aside in large bowl.

Place ¼ cup of the blueberries in blender with apple juice concentrate, dates, arrowroot, coriander, vanilla, and salt; blend until smooth. Pour this syrup over blueberries in bowl and mix well. Pour blueberry mixture into 13 x 9-inch baking dish.

Roll out pie dough into large oblong shape to cover pie (this will require plenty of counter space). Cover blueberries with dough. Tuck edges of dough just inside baking dish or flute edges against edge of dish, pressing to seal. Cut three small slits in crust to allow steam to escape.

Bake for 1 hour.   *Makes 12 to 15 servings*

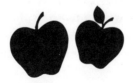

Deep-Dish Apple Pie

The sweetness in this apple pie comes from fruit concentrate and dates, not from sugar; therefore we do not recommend the tart or sour apples that are called for in sugar-filled pies. Use Golden Delicious apples so they can add their sweetness to the pie.

As with the previous recipe, the filling ingredients can be halved to make a double-crust 9-inch pie, or a deep-dish 9-inch pie covered with a single layer of pastry (half a recipe of Flaky Pie Crust).

12 Golden Delicious apples
1 can (12 ounces) frozen
    apple juice
    concentrate, thawed
1 cup pitted dates
¼ cup arrowroot

1 teaspoon ground
    coriander
1 teaspoon vanilla extract
½ teaspoon salt
1 recipe Flaky Pie Crust
    (page 44)

Preheat oven to 400°F.

Pare, core, and thinly slice apples. Place in large bowl.

Place in blender apple juice concentrate, dates, arrowroot, coriander, vanilla, and salt; blend until smooth. Mix this syrup with the apples and place in 13 x 9-inch baking dish.

Roll out pie dough into large oblong shape to cover pie (this will require plenty of counter space). Cover apple mixture with dough. Tuck edges of dough just inside baking dish or flute edges against edge of dish, pressing to seal. Cut three small slits in crust to allow steam to escape.

Bake for 1 hour.   *Makes 12 to 15 servings*

Deep-Dish Peach Pie

The peaches in this recipe tend to be so juicy that they are unsuitable for a round double-crust pie, but you can certainly halve the ingredients to make a deep-dish pie in an 8-inch square baking dish with a single covering crust.

10 cups thinly sliced
    peaches, fresh or
    frozen
1 can (12 ounces) frozen
    apple juice
    concentrate, thawed
1 cup pitted dates
¼ cup arrowroot

1 teaspoon ground
    coriander
½ teaspoon salt
½ teaspoon almond
    extract
1 recipe Flaky Pie Crust
    (page 44)

Preheat oven to 350°F.

Place sliced peaches in large bowl.

Place in blender apple juice concentrate, dates, arrowroot, coriander, salt, and almond extract; blend until smooth. Add this syrup to sliced peaches and mix thoroughly. Place peach mixture in 13 x 9-inch baking dish.

Roll out pie crust dough to large oblong and cover peaches. Tuck edges of dough just inside baking dish or flute edges against edge of dish, pressing to seal. Cut three small slits in crust to allow steam to escape.

Bake for 50 to 60 minutes.   *Makes 12 to 15 servings*

Orchard Apple-Peach Cobbler

Apples and peaches delicately flavored with almond make up this large cobbler.

If you want to make a double-crust pie with peaches, this is your recipe; peaches alone are too juicy for the double crust.

5 cups pared, cored, and sliced Golden Delicious apples	1 teaspoon ground coriander
6 cups sliced fresh peaches	¼ cup arrowroot
1 can (12 ounces) frozen apple juice concentrate, thawed	1 teaspoon vanilla extract
	½ teaspoon salt
	¼ teaspoon almond extract
1 cup pitted dates	1 recipe Flaky Pie Crust (page 44)

Preheat oven to 350°F.

Combine apples and peaches in large bowl.

Place in blender apple juice concentrate, dates, coriander, arrowroot, vanilla, salt, and almond extract; blend until smooth. Add this syrup to apples and peaches and mix thoroughly. Place mixture in 13 x 9-inch baking dish.

Roll out pie crust dough to large oblong, and cover fruit. Tuck edges of dough under just inside edge of baking dish or flute edges against dish, pressing to seal. Cut three small slits in crust to allow steam to escape.

Bake for 1 hour.   *Makes 12 to 15 servings*

Blueberry Crisp

This is a recipe to use when you want something convenient —fresh fruit requires little preparation and the topping here is easily made of granola.

5¼ cups fresh or frozen blueberries
1 can (6 ounces) frozen apple juice concentrate, thawed
½ cup pitted dates
2 tablespoons arrowroot
1 teaspoon ground coriander

1 teaspoon vanilla extract
¼ teaspoon salt
1 to 2 cups Sunrise Crunchy Granola (page 17) or other granola, preferably fruit-sweetened

Preheat oven to 350°F.

Wash blueberries and place in large bowl.

Place ¼ cup of the blueberries in blender with apple juice concentrate, dates, arrowroot, coriander, vanilla, and salt; blend until smooth. Pour this syrup over blueberries in bowl and gently stir. Put in 8-inch square baking dish and bake for 25 minutes.

Remove from oven and cover with granola. Return to oven and bake until bubbly, about 12 minutes more. (Watch carefully to make sure granola topping does not burn.)   ***Makes 10 servings***

Baked Pumpkin Pie

½ cup raw cashews, well rinsed
¾ cup water
1 cup pitted dates
1 cup boiling water
1½ cups pumpkin puree
¼ cup arrowroot
¼ cup honey
2 teaspoons ground coriander

1 teaspoon vanilla or maple extract
½ teaspoon orange extract
½ teaspoon salt
1 unbaked pie shell, made from Flaky Pie Crust recipe (page 44)

Preheat oven to 350°F.

Place cashews and ¾ cup water in blender and blend until very creamy. Remove from blender and place in bowl.

Put dates in blender. Pour boiling water over them and let stand while you assemble the remaining ingredients. Blend dates thoroughly. (With some blenders you must be very careful while blending hot ingredients. Try starting on low speed and cracking the lid just a bit if it's self-sealing.)

Add pumpkin and liquified cashews and blend. Add arrowroot, honey, coriander, extracts, and salt; blend again. (If your blender container is too small to handle all this, once the dates are processed you can transfer them to a bowl and mix the rest by hand.)

Pour filling into unbaked pie shell. Bake for 1 hour or until pie is almost set in center.   *Makes 8 servings*

Pineapple-Coconut Tarts

These tarts are flavorful and tart, *and those who love them love them with a passion.*

1 recipe Flaky Pie Crust
   dough (page 44)
3 cups fresh or
   unsweetened canned
   pineapple chunks,
   drained if canned
1 cup chopped pitted
   dates
1 cup raisins
½ cup finely shredded
   unsweetened coconut
1 can (6 ounces) frozen
   pineapple juice
   concentrate, thawed

1 teaspoon ground
   coriander
¼ teaspoon salt
¼ teaspoon lemon extract
1 tablespoon arrowroot
1 tablespoon water
1 teaspoon grated lemon
   peel
   Chopped nuts to garnish
   (optional)

Prepare tart shells: Preheat oven to 450°F. Roll pie crust dough into 15-inch circle on floured surface. Cut dough into ten 2-inch rounds; press rounds into wells of muffin tins. (It will be necessary to *press* dough outward with your fingers until it is very thin.) Prick bottom and sides of pastry shells thoroughly with fork to prevent puffing. Bake for 10 minutes. Cool before removing from pans.

Prepare filling: Cook pineapple chunks, dates, raisins, coconut, pineapple juice concentrate, coriander, salt, and extract in large saucepan over low heat until tender, stirring occasionally, approximately 15 minutes. Moisten arrowroot, stirring, with 1 tablespoon water; add to heated fruit and stir in gently. Cook over low heat until glaze is thickened and clear. Add grated lemon peel and stir in gently. Remove from heat and allow to cool.

Spoon filling into baked tart shells. Top with optional nuts as garnish. Serve warm or cool. ***Makes 10 servings***

Old-Fashioned Dutch Raisin Pie

This pie for raisin lovers is best when served slightly warm.

1 recipe Flaky Pie Crust
  (page 44)
2 cups raisins
¼ cup finely chopped
  pitted dates
2 cups water
¼ cup honey
1 teaspoon ground
  coriander

¼ cup arrowroot
½ cup chopped pecans
3 tablespoons fresh lemon
  juice
2 teaspoons grated lemon
  peel

Preheat oven to 400°F.

Roll out half of pie crust dough and line 9-inch pie plate.

Heat raisins, dates, and water to boiling in 2-quart saucepan; reduce heat and cook over low heat for 5 minutes. Stir in honey and coriander, then slowly add arrowroot. Stir constantly until mixture thickens and boils.

Remove from heat. Stir in chopped pecans, lemon juice, and lemon peel.

Pour hot filling into pastry-lined pie plate. Roll out top crust and cover filling; seal and flute edges. Cut two tiny slits in crust to allow steam to escape.

Bake for 30 minutes. ***Makes 8 to 10 servings***

Christmas Mince Pie

We have found that many people prefer this pie to traditional mince.

Though many of these recipes work much better with a blender, this is one recipe that requires a food processor or a food grinder for grinding the dates, raisins, prunes, and walnuts. Of course, it also requires a blender for emulsifying the oil and water for the pie crust! Delicious as it is, this pie is a bit of a production that calls for an occasion like Christmas —or a visit from a favored friend whose favorite pie is mince.

1 recipe Flaky Pie Crust
   (page 44)
1 can (6 ounces) frozen
   apple juice
   concentrate, thawed
3 tablespoons arrowroot
2 tablespoons fresh lemon
   juice
1 teaspoon grated lemon
   peel

1 teaspoon ground
   coriander
1 teaspoon vanilla extract
1 cup pitted dates
1 cup raisins
½ cup pitted prunes
½ cup chopped walnuts
2 cups peeled, cored, and
   coarsely shredded
   apples

Preheat oven to 375°F.

Line 9-inch pie plate with half of pie crust dough.

Place in blender apple juice concentrate, arrowroot, lemon juice, lemon peel, coriander, and vanilla; blend until smooth. Set aside.

Place in food processor pitted dates, raisins, pitted prunes, and walnuts and process until finely ground; or process through a food grinder. Set aside.

Place apples in large bowl. Add apple juice mixture and ground fruit mixture and mix well.

Pour fruit mixture into pastry-lined pie plate. Roll out top crust and cover fruit mixture; seal and crimp edges. Cut two tiny slits in crust to allow steam to escape.

Bake for 45 minutes.   ***Makes 8 to 10 servings***

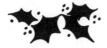

Banana Date-Nut Cookies

*These cookies are very sweet and flavorful and have a pleas-
ant texture.*

3 medium-size very ripe
   bananas, mashed
2 cups rolled oats
1 cup chopped pecans
1 cup chopped pitted
   dates

⅓ cup frozen orange juice
   concentrate, thawed
¼ cup canola oil
½ teaspoon almond extract
½ teaspoon salt

Preheat oven to 300°F.

Mix all ingredients thoroughly in large bowl and let stand approximately 5 minutes to absorb moisture.

Drop cookies by large spoonfuls onto lightly oiled baking sheets,
spacing 1 inch apart.

Bake for 30 minutes or until golden brown.

Makes approximately 2½ dozen cookies

Orange Date-Nut Cake

*This is a healthful substitute for a traditional fruitcake,
rather heavy and sweet—but most people we have served it to
like it much better than the traditional fruitcake. It is wonderful served with Orange-Pineapple Sauce (page 41) or with
Tangy Sweet Lemon Sauce (page 40). Use the larger amounts
of lemon juice in these recipes, as the cake itself is very sweet.*

2 cups chopped walnuts
1½ cups chopped pitted
   dates
1½ cups chopped raisins
1 cup whole-wheat pastry
   flour
½ cup frozen orange juice
   concentrate, thawed
½ cup Date Butter (recipe
   follows)

2 tablespoons canola oil
1 teaspoon almond
   extract
½ teaspoon orange
   extract
1 teaspoon grated orange
   peel
½ teaspoon salt

Preheat oven to 300°F.

Mix together in large bowl walnuts, dates, raisins, and flour (it may be necessary to use your hands).

In second bowl, mix together orange juice concentrate, Date Butter, oil, almond and orange extracts, orange peel, and salt. Add to walnut-date mixture and mix thoroughly.

Place mixture in lightly oiled 9 x 5 x 3-inch loaf pan or Bundt pan. Press evenly into pan.

Bake for 50 to 60 minutes. **Makes 12 servings**

Date Butter

Besides using Date Butter in baking cakes such as Orange Date-Nut Cake, Adventists use it in hot cereal and as a spread for toast or peanut-butter bread.

1 cup pitted dates **½ cup boiling water**

Place pitted dates in blender. Pour boiling water over dates, cover, and let stand 10 minutes. (With some blenders you must be careful while blending hot ingredients. Either let the water cool for longer than 10 minutes, begin blending at low speed, and/or crack the top of a close-fitting lid.)

Blend until smooth. **Makes approximately 1 cup**

Chewy Granola Bars

No collection of healthy sweets would be complete without a recipe for flavorful granola bars!

It's best to use your fingers to combine the peanut-butter mixture with the dry ingredients, working the mixture till it has the texture of fine crumbs.

¼ cup honey
½ cup natural crunchy
  peanut butter
2 teaspoons vanilla
  extract
2 cups whole-wheat
  pastry flour
1½ cups rolled oats
½ cup oat bran

½ cup chopped pecans
⅓ cup finely shredded
  unsweetened coconut
¼ cup sunflower seeds
1 teaspoon coriander
1 teaspoon salt
1½ cups chopped pitted
  dates
¼ cup water, if necessary

Preheat oven to 350°F.

Soften honey and peanut butter in small saucepan over low heat, stirring well. Stir in vanilla. Remove from heat.

Thoroughly mix flour, oats, oat bran, pecans, coconut, seeds, coriander, and salt in large bowl. Add peanut butter–honey mixture and mix lightly until completely moistened and crumbly. Add dates. If mixture seems too dry to press into baking pan, sprinkle with water until moistened.

Press mixture firmly into lightly oiled 13 x 9-inch baking dish. Bake for 15 to 20 minutes or until toasty.

Cool and cut into bars.   ***Makes approximately 2 dozen bars***

Peanut Butter Crunchies

Somewhere between a cookie and a fudge, these are always a favorite. The key is to make sure not to overbake, or the Crunchies will become dry very quickly. Watch the batter carefully until the edges barely darken, then quickly take the pan out of the oven.

½ cup whole-wheat pastry
  flour
½ cup Sunrise Crunchy
  Granola (page 17) or
  other granola,
  preferably fruit-
  sweetened
2 tablespoons finely
  shredded unsweetened
  coconut

½ cup natural crunchy
  peanut butter
¼ cup honey
2 tablespoons canola oil
1 teaspoon vanilla extract
⅛ teaspoon salt
¼ teaspoon lemon extract
½ teaspoon ground
  coriander (optional)

Preheat oven to 350°F.

Mix together flour, granola, and coconut and set aside.

Mix remaining ingredients well, then add dry ingredients and combine thoroughly. (You may need to warm the peanut butter in a saucepan over low heat until it is soft enough to work with a spoon, then stir in the remaining ingredients as instructed.) Place batter in 8-inch square baking dish, patting down the top.

Bake for 10 to 12 minutes (or even less), just till edges begin to turn brown. Remove from oven, cool, and cut into bars.

Makes 12 to 16 bars

Holiday Fudgeless Fudgies

This is the first of a concentrated fudgy quartet that is dreamy and delicious. Though much more healthful than traditional fudges, these treats are concentrated in calories. Bring out these recipes at holiday time!

In making all these candies, you will need to get physical. Use your hands!

½ cup natural crunchy peanut butter
½ cup honey
1 teaspoon ground coriander
1 teaspoon vanilla extract
½ cup raw sunflower seeds
½ cup roasted carob powder

½ cup raisins
¼ cup chopped pecans
¼ cup unhulled sesame seeds
2 tablespoons finely shredded unsweetened coconut

Heat peanut butter, honey, coriander, and vanilla in a large saucepan over low heat until softened. Stir until smooth.

Remove from heat and mix in remaining ingredients until thoroughly moistened. You may knead mixture with your hands.

Press mixture firmly and evenly into lightly oiled 8-inch square baking dish. Cover with plastic wrap and chill at least a few hours before cutting into squares approximately 1 to 2 inches in size.

Makes 2 dozen squares

Almond Butter Carob Fudge

½ cup almond butter
¼ cup honey
2 tablespoons oil
¼ teaspoon almond
    extract
¼ teaspoon orange
    extract
⅛ teaspoon salt
½ cup whole-wheat
    pastry flour

¼ cup granola,
    preferably fruit-
    sweetened
¼ cup sliced almonds
¼ cup carob chips
    (sweetened with
    dates or barley
    malt)

Preheat oven to 350°F.

Mix together almond butter, honey, oil, and extracts. Add salt, flour, granola, almonds, and carob chips. Mix well.

Press into 8-inch square baking dish. Bake for 12 to 15 minutes, just until edges turn slightly brown. Cool and cut into squares.

Makes 16 squares

Natural Nutty Chunkies

2 cups carob chips
    (sweetened with dates
    or barley malt)
¼ cup natural crunchy
    peanut butter
½ cup soy milk

1 teaspoon vanilla extract
⅛ teaspoon salt
1 cup raisins
½ cup chopped nuts
¼ cup finely shredded
    unsweetened coconut

Place carob chips in 2-quart saucepan and heat over low heat, stirring gently and constantly until chips begin to melt. Add peanut butter and continue to heat, stirring well. Add soy milk, vanilla, and salt, stirring and heating. Add raisins, nuts, and coconut, and mix thoroughly. Remove from heat.

Press mixture firmly and evenly into lightly oiled 11½ x 8-inch baking dish. Cover with plastic wrap and chill approximately 3 hours or until firm.

Cut into squares (it may be necessary to let candy sit out until it is soft enough to cut). *Makes 2 dozen 2-inch squares*

Chewy Moroccan Carob Balls

Buy crispy brown rice—the healthy, sugarless version of crispy rice cereal—at your local health food store. Try dried pineapple, figs, dates, or other dried fruit in this recipe.

You can make the granola crumbs by placing granola in the blender or food processor and blending thoroughly.

1 cup natural crunchy peanut butter	½ cup chopped nuts
½ cup honey	½ cup finely chopped dried fruit
1 teaspoon vanilla extract	Granola crumbs, approximately ½ cup
½ cup crispy brown rice	
½ cup roasted carob powder	

Soften peanut butter and honey in large saucepan over low heat, stirring. Stir in vanilla.

Add remaining ingredients (except granola crumbs) and mix well. Remove from heat.

Form into 1-inch balls and roll in granola crumbs. Chill approximately 3 hours until firm.　　**Makes approximately 2½ dozen**

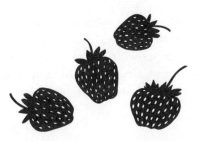

Strawberry Fruit Smoothie

Everybody loves fruit smoothies, and you can make them with just about any fruit. Frozen bananas are standard because of the sweetness and texture they add, but if you don't like bananas, substitute other frozen fruit. (You can also add ice cubes, if your blender is powerful enough to handle them.) If your combination of fruit is not quite sweet enough, add a little honey. Experiment with other flavorings as well, such as vanilla or almond extract.

3 medium-size ripe
   bananas, frozen
1 cup fresh strawberries
1 cup fresh or unsweetened
   canned pineapple
   chunks, drained if
   canned

1 cup melon or other
   summer fruit chunks
1 cup orange juice
1 cup unsweetened
   pineapple juice
1 teaspoon ground
   coriander

Cut bananas into large chunks and place in blender. Add rest of ingredients and blend until smooth.

Pour into tall glasses.   *Makes 8 servings*

Peppermint Cooler

This is the first of several nonalcoholic coolers that feature unbeatable combinations of herb teas, fruits, and juices.

Most of these beverage recipes make a fairly large amount —you may, of course, halve the recipes if you want to make a smaller amount.

For a less sweet or concentrated drink, you can also add more water for all the recipes. Jan prefers to add more honey or less water for a sweeter drink. You may thaw the juice concentrates before mixing and add cold water—or leave the concentrates partially frozen, thawed just enough for mixing.

2 cups boiling water
4 peppermint tea bags
   Honey to taste
2 cups cold water
1 can (12 ounces) frozen
   pineapple juice
   concentrate, thawed
1 can (12 ounces) frozen
   orange juice
   concentrate, thawed

1 can (12 ounces) frozen
   apple juice
   concentrate, thawed
2 medium-size ripe
   bananas

Make iced tea: Pour boiling water over tea bags and let steep 4 to 6 minutes. Remove tea bags, stir in optional honey (usually 1 teaspoon per cup), and add cold water. Mix well and chill.

Mix juice concentrates in large pitcher or punch bowl, using 2 cans of water for each can of concentrate instead of the usual 3. Pour 2 cups of juice into blender with bananas and blend until smooth.

Add blended mixture and peppermint tea to juices and stir.

Makes 20 servings

Frosty Mint Delight

2 cups boiling water
4 mint tea bags
   Honey to taste
2 cups cold water
1 can (12 ounces) frozen
   pineapple juice
   concentrate, thawed
1 can (12 ounces) frozen
   apple juice
   concentrate, thawed

1 can (6 ounces) frozen
   grapefruit juice
   concentrate, thawed
2 medium-size ripe
   bananas, frozen
1 teaspoon ground
   coriander

Make iced tea: Pour boiling water over tea bags and let steep for 4 to 6 minutes. Remove tea bags, stir in honey (usually 1 teaspoon per cup), and add cold water. Mix well and chill.

Mix juice concentrates in large pitcher or punch bowl, using 2 cans of water per can of concentrate instead of the usual 3. Pour 2 cups of juice into blender.

Add cut-up bananas and coriander to juice in blender and blend until smooth. Add blended mixture and mint tea to juices in pitcher and stir.

Makes 15 to 20 servings

The Amen Special

Chris named this drink after she served it to one of the stars of the hit television series "Amen." Clifton Davis was a guest in her home when she concocted a fruit drink using the grapefruit juice she had on hand. Mr. Davis took one sip, put the drink down with a startled look, and said, "What's in this? I can't drink this!" He had given up alcohol several years before and had no intention of taking it up again. Chris at last convinced him there was no alcohol in the drink, though he insisted: "I used to have a cocktail that tasted just like this every day!"

1 can (12 ounces) frozen
    pineapple juice
    concentrate, thawed
1 can (12 ounces) frozen
    orange juice
    concentrate, thawed
1 can (12 ounces) frozen
    apple juice
    concentrate, thawed

1 can (6 ounces) frozen
    grapefruit juice
    concentrate, thawed
2 medium-size ripe
    bananas, frozen
1 cup sweet cantaloupe
    chunks
1 teaspoon ground
    coriander

Place juice concentrates in large punch bowl, add 2 to 3 cans of water per can of concentrate and stir thoroughly (the smaller amount of water will result in a sweeter drink). Pour 2 cups of the juice into blender.

Add cut-up frozen bananas, cantaloupe, and coriander to juice in blender and blend until smooth. Add blended mixture to punch bowl and stir well. Serve on the rocks and chill out!

Makes 15 to 20 servings

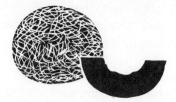

Zingy Lemon Rush

For Red Zinger Holiday Fruit Punch, substitute Red Zinger tea for the Lemon Zinger tea.

2 cups boiling water
4 Lemon Zinger tea bags
    Up to ¼ cup honey
    (optional)

2 cups cold water
1 can (12 ounces) frozen
    apple juice
    concentrate, thawed

1 can (12 ounces) frozen
   orange juice
   concentrate, thawed
1 can (12 ounces) frozen
   pineapple juice
   concentrate, thawed

2 medium-size ripe
   bananas
1 teaspoon ground
   coriander

Make iced tea: Pour boiling water over tea bags and let steep 4 to 6 minutes. Remove tea bags, stir in optional honey, and add cold water. Mix well and chill.

Mix juice concentrates in large pitcher or punch bowl, using 2 cans of water per can of concentrate instead of the usual 3. Pour 2 cups of the juice into blender.

Add cut-up bananas and coriander to juice in blender and blend until smooth. Add blended mixture and Lemon Zinger tea to juices in pitcher and stir.   ***Makes 20 servings***

Orange Rush

1 can (12 ounces) frozen
   unsweetened orange
   juice concentrate,
   thawed
1 can (12 ounces) frozen
   unsweetened pineapple
   juice concentrate,
   thawed

1 can (12 ounces) frozen
   unsweetened apple
   juice concentrate,
   thawed
2 medium-size ripe
   bananas
1 teaspoon ground
   coriander

Place juice concentrates in a pitcher or punch bowl and mix with water as directed on cans. (For a sweeter drink, add less water.)

Place bananas in blender and add coriander and a cup or two of the mixed juices. Blend until smooth.

Add banana mixture to juices, stir, and serve.

      Makes about 5 quarts

Strawberry-Tropical Punch

1 can (12 ounces) frozen
    pineapple juice
    concentrate, thawed
1 can (12 ounces) frozen
    apple juice
    concentrate, thawed
1 can (12 ounces) frozen
    orange juice
    concentrate, thawed
2 medium-size ripe
    bananas
2 cups fresh or frozen
    unsweetened
    strawberries
1 teaspoon ground
    coriander

Mix juice concentrates in large pitcher or punch bowl, using 2 to 3 cans of water per can of concentrate and stir thoroughly (the smaller amount of water will make sweeter drink). Pour 2 cups of the juice into blender.

Add cut-up banana(s), strawberries, and coriander to juice in blender and blend until smooth. Add blended mixture to juices in pitcher and stir.   *Makes 15 to 20 servings*

January Zingy Lemon Tea

4 cups water
4 Lemon Zinger tea bags
    Honey to taste
1 can (12 ounces) frozen
    orange juice
    concentrate, thawed
1 can (12 ounces) frozen
    apple juice
    concentrate, thawed
1 teaspoon ground
    coriander
¼ teaspoon lemon extract

Make hot tea: Boil water in large saucepan and add tea bags; let steep for 4 to 6 minutes. Remove tea bags and stir in honey (usually 1 teaspoon per cup), juice concentrates, 2 to 3 cans water per can of concentrate, coriander, and lemon extract.

Bring to a simmer and serve hot.   *Makes 15 servings*

Apple Zinger Iced Tea

4 cups boiling water
8 Red Zinger tea bags
   Honey to taste
4 cups cold water

1 can (12 ounces) frozen
   apple juice
   concentrate, thawed
½ cup fresh lemon juice

Make iced tea: Pour boiling water over tea bags and let steep 4 to 6 minutes. Remove tea bags, stir in optional honey. Add cold water. Mix well and chill.

Add undiluted apple juice concentrate and lemon juice and stir well.   *Makes 10 servings*

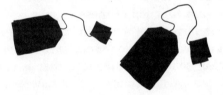

. W O R K I N G   T H E .
P R O G R A M

It is a delightful surprise to discover that the dessert and beverage recipes in this chapter are as wonderfully sweet and flavorful as any recipes loaded with sugar and the "bad" kind of fat! If your family is in the habit of eating sugary desserts, slip them a slice of Blueberry Pie or Apple-Peach Cobbler to preserve their health.

However—as healthful as concentrated fruit juices, nuts, and dried fruits are, they are still concentrated foods. This means they should be used more sparingly than the plain fruits, vegetables, whole grains, and legumes.

In fact, if your goal is rapid weight loss, it might be best to savor most of these delicious desserts through a careful *reading* of the recipes!

So why, then, present these recipes at all? They have absolutely no cholesterol, and very little saturated fat—so if your weight is not a concern and you are mainly interested in controlling your cholesterol intake, you may indulge in these treats from time to time with a clear conscience.

Once a week Chris makes a special dessert for her family—a cobbler or a deep-dish pie. She prepares it to be eaten on the Sabbath, a day of worship, resting, and fellowship, with the companionship of family and friends. Undoubtedly you have your own special occasions that would be enhanced by a special dessert, and it's always nice to have recipes for candies and refreshing drinks for holidays and parties.

The desserts in this chapter are also perfect for guests who expect dessert, especially those who are skeptical of your ability to make healthful desserts that taste good. Go ahead—serve Summer Fresh Fruit Pie or Blueberry Crisp—and knock 'em out!

Another important function of these recipes is winning over your children. If yours have a sweet tooth, try giving them Pineapple-Orange Sherbet or Peach Cobbler or one of the other desserts. Knowing they're getting some good nutrition that is entirely lacking in sugar-filled desserts, you'll acquire a little more peace of mind—and your child will love them!

After the novelty of "health" cobblers and pies has died down, you will find that for daily fare whole fresh fruits are best. A bowl of colorful apples, oranges, pears, or grapes makes a beautiful centerpiece and a tasty and wholesome end to a meal.

It has become a part of nutritional lore that "honey is as bad as sugar." Well, it's not quite as bad, and we see no problem with its sparing use to help sweeten herb teas and the occasional dessert. It may also be used in an emergency, to drizzle the fruits you have bought for an important meal if you discover they are not quite as sweet as required.

Even better as sweeteners are dried fruits and fruit concentrates, which have more vitamins and minerals than does honey. Dried fruits have the additional bonus of fiber. Some people don't like dates, but when blended dates are used to sweeten a dessert, it is their sweetness and not their flavor that you taste.

Most of the desserts in this chapter are *very* sweet. Your ultimate goal, of course, is to train your palate so that the natural sweetness of fresh fruit is enough. But this will happen gradually. The average sugar-trained palate will welcome the sweetness of these desserts.

After a while you may wish to cut back on the amount of honey used in the recipes, first trying two-thirds the specified amount, then half. You may also control the sweetness of date-sweetened desserts by using fewer dates.

Can you give up sugar? Some report that it's difficult at first, because sugar gives them a lift that is so irresistible that the longing for it resembles a kind of addiction. It may be easier to "tough it out," to cut out sugar completely, than to simply cut back on it. Once the cravings subside (and they will), most people find that they feel better than they did when they relied on sugar to give them temporary lifts throughout the day.

Another important step in cutting out empty and refined calories is switching to whole grains. Some people think they don't like whole-grain bread, but there are so many kinds on the market now we are sure you will find one that will appeal to you. Not only is it best to eat a variety of whole grains—millet, oats, barley, etc.—but in see-through canisters, they make a nice addition to your kitchen decor.

Throughout this book we recommend that you make changes gradually. Some people are convinced that they can't digest whole grains and seeds—not to mention beans! It is especially important to add these foods to your diet a little at a time. The reward comes when your body adjusts to these foods and begins to function the way it was meant to, helping you to maintain an appropriate weight and a healthy body.

· S U M M A R Y ·

1. If you are trying to lose weight, more important than cutting back on the quantity of food you eat is improving the quality of your food by cutting out empty and refined calories.

2. The alarming rise in the development of chronic degenerative disease (including obesity) is one result of the increasing production and consumption of refined and processed foods.

3. Almost 60 percent of the daily American diet is made up of refined and empty calories, providing virtually no nutrition, and ending up as body fat on the consumer.

4. To reverse this trend in your own life, acquiring health and slim-

ness along the way, eat a variety of whole natural vegetables, fruits, grains, beans, and nuts.

• This Week's Guide to Success •

Leave out refined foods when planning your meals.

These include white bread, white macaroni, white rice, refined breakfast cereals, instant potatoes, etc.

Include complex carbohydrates in your meals.

These include whole-grain cereals, pasta, and breads, and brown rice.

Satisfy your sweet tooth the natural way with fresh fruits.

For an occasional special dessert, try a recipe from this chapter.

Begin to read the labels of the food items you are about to place in your shopping cart.

Try to avoid food products that are largely made up of refined ingredients.

3

· *Principle No. 3* ·

Increase Fruits and Vegetables

All should be acquainted with the special
value of fruits and vegetables fresh from the
orchard and garden.
—*Ellen G. White*

Believe it or not, the answer to the fat problem grows on trees
—it's not found in bottles of gaily colored pills! It droops from
the fruit-laden boughs of apple, pear, and peach trees. It buds from
heads of green cabbage and frosty white cauliflower, and is found in
vine-ripened tomatoes and slopes of golden cantaloupes. Principle
No. 3—increase fruits and vegetables—will enable you to begin to
experience the buoyancy of vibrant health. It promises greater vigor
and a trim, shapely new profile. So why do we look with disdain on
crisp, crinkly greens and tangy-sweet nectarines? Every voluntary
and official health agency tells us we should consume a minimum of
four servings of fruits and vegetables per day. Yet the average American eats a mere pittance of this share.

Sad to say, over 80 percent of our daily calories come from meat
and dairy products, visible fats, sugar, syrup, and refined breads and
cereals. A meager 8 percent comes from fruits and vegetables. Yet
from that lean amount comes 70 percent of our vitamin C and 49.7
percent of our vitamin A. If fruits and vegetables were increased
to make up 50 percent of the total calories, the vitamin and mineral
supply in our diet would increase six times. Studies across the board
suggest that our risk for developing chronic degenerative diseases
would drop dramatically if we incorporated this simple measure
into our life-style. For example, a study of more than six hundred
women conducted by the National Cancer Institute found that the
incidence of mouth and throat cancers declined as fruit and vege-

table consumption increased. The lowest risk was found in women who ate three or more servings of fruits and vegetables daily. The American Cancer Society and the National Cancer Institute make this recommendation: Eat more vegetables and fruits, two servings a day of each. That makes a minimum of four daily servings. A more recent recommendation from the National Academy of Sciences is that everyone eat *five* servings of fruits and vegetables daily.

Not only are fruits and vegetables underrepresented in our daily diet, but those we do eat may run a nutritional obstacle course through the modern processing ingenuity of refinement. Before reaching our stomachs, these life-giving foods are often mortified by being sterilized, dehydrated, irradiated, smoked, pickled, blanched, canned, and cooked, cooked, cooked!

The refining process tends to concentrate the valueless ingredients in foods—ingredients such as white flour, sugar, and shortening—adding more calories while subtracting nutrition. One cup of fresh sliced peaches is only 65 calories, but becomes 200 refined calories when canned with sugar. A delicious apple packed with natural sweetness is only 70 calories. Refined and concentrated into apple juice, it increases to 120 calories. Refine it into a slice of all-American apple pie and you have 350 calories. A plain baked potato has only a hundred calories. However, a serving of French fries pushes up the calories to 300. Hashbrowns soaked in animal fat soar to 400 calories, and a serving of potato chips (based on the same weight as the hash browns) peaks at a staggering 800 calories. Refining and concentrating our foods gives us fat bodies with decaying organs!

As you begin to use whole natural foods in your cooking, the dieter's fantasy of getting to eat as much as you want without gaining may well turn out not to be fantasy after all! So dream on, for every scrumptious bite of fresh vegetables, luscious fruits, and savory legumes contains a solution to the fat problem—and that is *fiber*. This is the term used to describe the parts of plants that your body does not digest. Generally, fiber passes through your system whole. But don't think it hasn't accomplished its fat-liberating mission. Fiber is weight management's best friend. The fibers in fruits and vegetables seem to slink calories right out of your body. In a research study by nutritionist June Kelsay, Ph.D., at Beltsville Human Nutrition Research Center, men placed on a high-fiber diet of fruits and vegetables excreted 150 calories per day more than men on a fiber-deficient diet of equal calories. And Dr. Kenneth Heaton of Britain's University of Bristol reported how he and his wife experienced apparently effortless weight loss as they increased their fiber intake.

Most high-fiber foods are of a low caloric density. A major finding in a research study revealed that when foods more concentrated in calories (high caloric density) were consumed, many more calories were ingested than when eating an even larger volume of low-caloric-density foods. The people consuming the low-caloric-density foods felt satisfied while consuming half as many calories. What are low-caloric-density foods? *Fruits and Vegetables.* Because they are generally high in fiber and water, you can feast on fruits and vegetables without taking in many calories. And looking in the mirror, you'll see the fat shrink away day by day!

What are high-caloric-density foods? They are the refined, high-fat, highly concentrated foods that, as we have seen, compose 86 percent of the American daily diet. Compare a 6-ounce steak with a cup of kidney beans. When placed side by side, their volume looks comparable—but what a difference in the density of those calories! The steak contains 660 calories, while the kidney beans contain only 250—and in the kidney beans are almost 10 grams of dietary fiber, while none are supplied in the steak. Guess how many heads of lettuce you would have to eat to take in 660 calories. Twenty-five!

If you want to win the battle against fat, fruits and vegetables will be your greatest allies. In Table 7 you can see how many servings of low-caloric-density vegetables you would have to ingest to reach only 510 calories. If you were on a 1,000-calorie diet, you would need to consume *twice* this amount each day. We're not recommending that you try! But the lesson is: You can eat a superabundance of fruits and vegetables and still lose weight.

Table 7 • *Nutrient Content of Selected Vegetables and Fruits*

Nutrients	2 cups grated carrots 6 cups string beans 8 cups summer squash	30 peaches
Calories	510	1050
Protein	30 g	30 g
Calcium	868 mg	270 g
Iron	12.8 mg	15 mg
Vitamin A	74,840 I.U.	39,600 I.U.
Thiamine	1.46 mg	0.6 mg
Riboflavin	2.06 mg	1.5 mg
Niacin	17.8 mg	30 mg
Vitamin C	276 mg	210 mg

If you were convinced that feasting on luscious fruits, crisp vegetables, and flavorful beans could help you lower your cholesterol as
well as lose weight, wouldn't you want to join the feast of nature's
delights? Researchers feel that fiber serves as a vehicle to remove
excess bile acids and cholesterol, which would otherwise be recycled
and further increase cholesterol buildup. Remember, the final burial
ground for much of the body's excess cholesterol is the arteries. A
high-fiber diet can decrease your risk of a heart attack, and the best
sources of the kinds of fibers that lower serum cholesterol are apples,
beans, and oats.

If you were to replace empty and refined-calorie foods with fresh
fruits and vegetables, whole grains, beans, and nuts, you could say
farewell to unsightly fat! The satiety value of these whole foods alone
is a powerful weight-control measure. Principle No. 3—increase
fruits and vegetables—will give you some powerful ammunition for
the battle ahead. How much do we recommend? At least 4 to 6 servings—the more the better! It's the best health insurance you can
have. To get you started, here are some recipes to delight your
tastebuds.

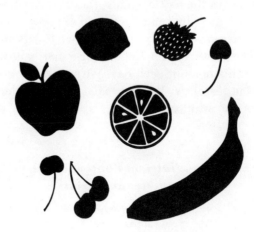

· R E C I P E S ·

Garden Patch Potato Stack

We decided to kick off the vegetable recipes with this one because we hope you will make it often! Chris eats it once a week!

Some of its virtues? It's a meal in itself. It's easy. And it's an absolutely delicious way to take in a large amount of the raw vegetables that are excellent for your health.

You may be surprised at what a massive amount of food it appears to make. This is because it is largely made of low-density raw vegetables. For most appetites, it will be just the right amount of food to make a substantial meal for four.

Pimiento Cashew Cheese seems to be everyone's favorite for this recipe, but you may also try it with Sunflower Pimiento Cheese or Hummus.

4 large potatoes, baked
    Vege-Sal or salt to taste
2 cups corn kernels, cut
    fresh from the cob
2 cups chopped tomatoes
1 bunch green onions,
    chopped
1 red bell pepper, cored,
    seeded, and chopped

2 cups shredded leaf or
    romaine lettuce
2 cups alfalfa sprouts
1 small ripe avocado,
    peeled, pitted, and
    sliced
1 cup shredded carrots
2 cups Pimiento Cashew
    Cheese (page 135)

Place freshly baked potatoes on individual plates. Slit them open and mash lightly. Sprinkle with Vege-Sal or salt.

Layer raw vegetables over potatoes (they will spill over sides of potatoes, forming large stacks on the plates). Top generously with Pimiento Cashew Cheese.

Dig in!   *Makes 4 servings*

Spinach Falafel

Use this recipe as a guide to making wonderful vegetable fillings for pita sandwiches. Fresh, natural ingredients in a combination such as this one always seem to enhance one another!

If you don't want to take the time to cook dried garbanzo beans, use canned, drained garbanzos.

1 bunch fresh spinach, washed, stemmed, and coarsely chopped
½ cup chopped black olives
½ cucumber, peeled if waxed, and chopped
½ green bell pepper, cored, seeded, and chopped
1 bunch green onions, chopped
½ cup chopped fresh mushrooms

½ cup cooked garbanzo beans
2 cups chopped tomatoes
1 cup chopped avocado
Cashonnaise (page 137) to moisten
Salt to taste
Whole-wheat pita breads
Alfalfa sprouts for garnish

Lightly mix together all ingredients except pita bread and sprouts, using enough Cashonnaise to moisten.

Stuff mixture into pita pockets and garnish with alfalfa sprouts.

Makes 4 to 6 pita pockets

Nutty Baked Acorn Squash

Here is a delicious and simple way to serve this nutritious vegetable without drowning it in butter and brown sugar.

Choose squash that are not too large, so that you will be able to cover the baking dish.

2 medium-size acorn
squash
½ cup unsweetened
crushed pineapple,
undrained
⅓ cup chopped pecans

⅓ cup chopped pitted
dates
1 tablespoon honey
1 teaspoon ground
coriander
½ teaspoon salt

Preheat oven to 400°F.

Wash squash and cut in half. Remove seeds and fibers and place cavity side up in an ungreased baking dish.

Thoroughly combine remaining ingredients. Divide the mixture evenly among the squash halves.

Pour water into dish to depth of ¼ inch. Cover and bake for 30 minutes or until tender. *Makes 4 servings*

Vegetarian Delight

This delicious vegetable dish is too hearty to place on the side of the dinner plate. Serve it as a meal!

1 cup raw brown rice
2 cups cauliflower florets
2 cups broccoli florets
1 recipe Southern-Style
Gravy (page 141)
1 package natural
mushroom soup mix

1 cup small mushroom
caps
1 medium-size onion,
thinly sliced

Prepare rice according to package directions.

While rice is cooking, prepare vegetables: Bring 1 inch of water to boil in large saucepan. Place cauliflower and broccoli in stainless-steel steamer basket and place basket in pan. Cover tightly. Turn heat down to low and steam until vegetables are crisp-tender, 7 to 10 minutes.

Prepare Southern-Style Gravy according to instructions. Just after it has begun to thicken, add mushroom soup mix, mushroom caps, and sliced onion. Simmer over medium-low heat for 5 minutes, stirring occasionally.

Add cauliflower and broccoli to gravy and serve over brown rice.

Makes 3 to 4 servings

Eastern Vegan Sauté

These vegetables are best served fresh out of the pan.

While cooking, keep the heat on high so vegetables will stay crispy. Stir constantly so they will cook evenly.

The subtle flavors of the sesame oil, garlic, and soy sauce permit the natural goodness of the vegetables to come through. You may want to add more soy sauce, especially if you serve the sauté over rice.

1 tablespoon sesame oil
3 cups thinly sliced Savoy
    cabbage
1 cup matchstick-cut
    carrots
½ cup finely chopped leeks

½ cup thinly sliced celery,
    cut on the diagonal
2 cloves garlic, minced
¼ cup water
1 tablespoon soy sauce or
    to taste

Heat oil in large skillet or wok, just to point of fragrance. Add cabbage, carrots, leeks, celery, garlic, and water. Stir vegetables constantly with wooden spoon over high heat until crisp-tender, 4 to 5 minutes.

Add soy sauce and stir. Serve immediately. ***Makes 4 servings***

Oriental-Style Vegetable Medley

This is another recipe for those who love combinations of crisp-tender vegetables. Serve over brown rice and add soy sauce for flavor.

1 cup raw brown rice
1 tablespoon olive oil
3 cups shredded green
    cabbage
1 cup thinly, diagonally
    sliced celery
1 cup chopped leeks

1 green bell pepper,
    cored, seeded, and cut
    in thin diagonal slices
1 teaspoon Vege-Sal or ½
    teaspoon salt
¼ cup water
Soy sauce to taste

Prepare rice according to package directions.

While rice is cooking, heat oil in large saucepan over medium heat and add vegetables and Vege-Sal or salt. Stir constantly for 2 to 3 minutes, coating vegetables with oil.

Add water, cover saucepan immediately, and steam over low heat for 5 minutes or until vegetables are crisp-tender. Serve immediately, over rice. *Makes 4 servings*

Glorified Almond Cauliflower

1 medium-size head cauliflower, trimmed and washed	1 cup Cashonnaise (page 137)
	1 cup sliced almonds

Preheat oven to 350°F.

Bring 1 inch of water to boil in large saucepan. Place cauliflower head in stainless-steel steamer basket and place basket in pan. Cover tightly. Turn heat down to low and steam until cauliflower is crisp-tender, 12 to 15 minutes.

Remove cauliflower from steamer basket and place in 9-inch pie plate; add a little of the water used for steaming to bottom of pie plate.

Smooth thick coating of Cashonnaise over entire head of cauliflower; press almond slices into Cashonnaise to cover completely.

Bake for 5 to 10 minutes, just to heat through.

Makes 5 to 6 servings

Cauliflower Supreme

There are some good preservative-free bottled spaghetti sauces on the market. Leftover spaghetti sauce can be added to beans, soups, or other savory dishes.

1 large head cauliflower, washed and broken into florets	1 cup chopped green bell pepper
Vege-Sal to taste	2½ cups natural spaghetti sauce
1½ cups chopped leeks	1 cup shredded soy mozzarella
1 cup sliced mushrooms	

¼ cup whole-grain cracker crumbs, onion-flavored if possible	1 teaspoon Italian seasoning

Preheat oven to 350°F.

Bring 1 inch of water to boil in large saucepan. Place cauliflower florets in stainless-steel basket and place basket in pan. Cover tightly. Turn heat down to low and steam until florets are crisp-tender, 7 to 10 minutes.

Place florets in 11½ x 8-inch baking dish. Sprinkle lightly with Vege-Sal. Layer leeks, mushrooms, bell pepper, and spaghetti sauce over florets, in that order. Top with soy mozzarella and cracker crumbs. Sprinkle with Italian seasoning.

Bake for 15 minutes or until bubbly.   *Makes 5 to 6 servings*

Nature's Best Baked Corn

This traditional method produces sweeter corn than does boiling because the silk and husks retain the corn's sweet natural juices. When the corn is done, remove the husks and silk and serve hot.

It's an easy, delightful summer dish!

6 ears corn, unhusked

Preheat oven to 350°F.

Place corn on oven rack and bake in husks for 20 minutes or until husks are golden brown.   *Makes 6 servings*

Corn Tamale Casserole

This casserole is pungent with cumin and garlic and various vegetables in a cornmeal base. If you like, you may top it with some shredded soy cheddar or soy mozzarella for the last 15 minutes of baking.

1 cup stone-ground yellow cornmeal

1 cup whole-kernel corn, fresh or frozen, drained

1 cup sliced pitted black olives

2 cups chopped tomatoes

1 cup soy milk

1 cup chopped green onions

½ cup green bell pepper, cored, seeded, and chopped

¼ cup garbanzo flour or soy flour

1 teaspoon ground cumin

1 teaspoon dried sweet basil

1 teaspoon ground coriander

1½ teaspoons salt

1 teaspoon Bakon seasoning

1 teaspoon ground sage

½ teaspoon garlic powder

Paprika

Preheat oven to 350°F.

Combine all ingredients except paprika in a large bowl and mix well. Pour into an 11½ x 8-inch baking dish. Sprinkle with paprika. Bake for 50 to 60 minutes or until set. *Makes 8 servings*

Cashew Eggplant Bake

"I don't much care for eggplant," said one taster, "but this I like!"

To ensure a crisp and crunchy coating, you may turn on the broiler toward the end of cooking time and broil for a minute or two on each side, watching closely so it doesn't burn.

2 cups whole-grain cracker crumbs, onion-flavored if possible

2 medium-size eggplants, peeled and cut in ¼-inch slices

1 cup Cashonnaise (page 137)

Preheat oven to 350°F.

Place cracker crumbs on a plate or shallow bowl. Coat eggplant slices with Cashonnaise, using a knife to spread a thin layer. Dip them in cracker crumbs to coat.

Place breaded eggplant slices on lightly oiled baking dishes. Bake for 20 minutes, turning after 10 to 12 minutes, until golden brown on each side.   *Makes 4 to 6 servings*

Baked Eggplant Romany

This is a well-seasoned dish that eggplant lovers will acclaim! The eggplant slices are breaded and baked as for Cashew Eggplant Bake, but you may dip them in soy milk or coat them with one of the pimiento cheese sauces instead of Cashonnaise if you prefer.

2 large eggplants
½ to 1 cup Cashonnaise (page 137)
1 to 2 cups whole-grain cracker crumbs
2 tablespoons olive oil
¼ cup water
1 cup chopped onion
1 cup chopped green bell pepper
1 cup sliced mushrooms
1 cup chopped celery
1 jar (32 ounces) natural spaghetti sauce
1 teaspoon dried sweet basil

1 teaspoon ground coriander
1 teaspoon dried sage
1 teaspoon Vege-Sal or ½ teaspoon salt
½ teaspoon garlic powder
2 cups sliced summer squash
2 cups shredded soy mozzarella
2 cups chopped leeks
2 tablespoons whole-grain cracker crumbs
1 teaspoon Italian seasoning

Preheat oven to 350°F.

Peel eggplant and cut into ½-inch slices. Bread and bake according to the method given in the preceding recipe (Cashew Eggplant Bake).

While eggplant is baking, heat olive oil and water in large saucepan over medium heat. Add onions, bell pepper, mushrooms, and celery and sauté until vegetables are crisp-tender. Add spaghetti sauce, basil, coriander, sage, Vege-Sal or salt, and garlic powder to vegetables and simmer uncovered over low heat, stirring occasionally, for 10 to 15 minutes.

To sliced baked eggplant in 13 x 9-inch baking dish, add in layers the following: half of vegetable sauce mixture, 1 cup sliced summer squash, 1 cup soy cheese, and 1 cup chopped leeks. Make a single layer of remaining baked eggplant on top of soy cheese. Repeat layering of vegetable sauce, squash, cheese, and leeks. Top with a sprinkling of whole-grain cracker crumbs and Italian seasoning. Bake for 20 minutes. *Makes 8 to 10 servings*

Steamed Fresh Greens

There's no need to add animal fat when cooking greens; Bakon seasoning, a product derived from yeast, adds a meaty flavor without meat.

The cooking times given here are approximate. It is most important not to overcook, or the greens will lose their color and acquire an unpleasant texture.

1 pound greens (kale, mustard, beet tops, spinach, turnip, collards)
1 medium-size onion, finely chopped

2 teaspoons soy sauce
1 teaspoon olive oil
½ teaspoon Bakon seasoning

Remove imperfect leaves from greens. Wash greens several times in large bowl or sink of water, lifting greens out of water to allow sand to sink to bottom. Drain greens and cut into bite-size pieces.

Bring 1 inch of water to boil in large saucepan and place stainless-steel steamer basket in pan. Place cut greens in steamer basket, top with chopped onion, and sprinkle with soy sauce, olive oil, and Bakon seasoning, and toss lightly. Cover tightly, reduce heat to medium-high, and steam until greens are tender. For spinach or beet tops, steam 5 to 10 minutes. Mustard greens: 15 minutes. Collards or turnip greens: 20 minutes. Kale: 20 to 25 minutes.

Makes 2 to 3 servings

Stir-Fried Turnip Greens

This makes a visually stunning dish. Be sure to use the ripest deep-red tomatoes you can find, and make sure the greens are not steamed so long that they lose their own deep green color.

If you like, you may use spinach instead of turnip greens. Spinach will take less steaming time, about 5 to 10 minutes.

2 tablespoons olive oil
4 teaspoons soy sauce
2 pounds turnip greens, washed, trimmed, and cut into bite-size pieces
1 cup chopped leeks
1 cup chopped tomatoes
¼ cup water

Heat oil in wok or large skillet over medium-high heat. Add soy sauce, then greens, leeks, and tomatoes. Stir 2 to 3 minutes, coating greens with oil.

Add water, turn heat to low, cover, and steam for 12 to 15 minutes, stirring occasionally. Cover wok for last few minutes.

Makes 4 servings

Savory Potato Rounds

This is a delicious, simple way to prepare potatoes that children love.

The slices should be cut thin, less than ¼ inch thick.

2 to 3 medium-size Idaho or baking potatoes, unpeeled, scrubbed, and thinly sliced
Vege-Sal
Garlic powder
Onion powder
Paprika

Preheat broiler, placing rack 4 to 6 inches below broiling element.

Place potato slices in single layer on lightly oiled baking sheets. Sprinkle slices with small amount of Vege-Sal and garlic powder, and slightly larger amounts of onion powder and paprika. Place under broiler for approximately 5 minutes or until golden.

Remove from oven, turn slices over with a spatula, and sprinkle again with seasonings. Return to broil for another 5 minutes or so, or until golden.   ***Makes 4 to 6 servings***

Twice-Baked Au Gratin Potatoes

These potatoes are excellent as a main dish, served with a tossed salad, whole-grain bread, and a lightly steamed green vegetable. You may use an electric hand mixer to work the seasonings into the potatoes, or beat vigorously with a wooden spoon.

4 large potatoes, scrubbed and freshly baked	1 teaspoon Bakon seasoning (optional)
1 cup Pimiento Cashew Cheese (page 135)	1 cup chopped green onions
1 teaspoon dried sweet basil	1 cup chopped red bell pepper
1 teaspoon ground coriander	1 cup shredded soy cheddar
½ teaspoon salt	Paprika

Preheat oven to 350°F.

Slice into top of each baked potato; scoop out the inside, leaving thin shell. Place scooped-out portions of potatoes in a bowl and mash well. Add Pimiento Cashew Cheese, basil, coriander, salt, and Bakon seasoning, and beat vigorously. Stir in green onions and red bell pepper.

Fill each potato shell with one-fourth of the potato-vegetable mixture. Top with soy cheese and sprinkle lightly with paprika.

Bake for 15 minutes or until golden brown.   ***Makes 4 servings***

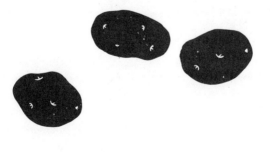

Creamy Scalloped Potatoes

This delicious dish may serve as a side dish or as an entrée.

1 recipe Pimiento Cashew Cheese (page 135)
2 teaspoons dried sweet basil
1 teaspoon ground coriander
1 teaspoon Vege-Sal or ½ teaspoon salt
1 teaspoon Bakon seasoning (optional)

8 medium-large potatoes, baked
1 bunch green onions, chopped
1 red bell pepper, cored, seeded, and chopped
1 cup shredded soy mozzarella
1 teaspoon paprika

Preheat oven to 350°F.

Blend Pimiento Cashew Cheese with basil, coriander, Vege-Sal or salt, and optional Bakon seasoning.

Peel baked potatoes and cut in slices ¼ to ½ inch in width. Place half the slices in lightly oiled 13 x 9-inch baking dish. On top of potatoes layer half the onions, red bell pepper, and seasoned Pimiento Cashew Cheese. Repeat layers with the remaining potatoes, onions, bell pepper, and seasoned Pimiento Cashew Cheese. Top with soy mozzarella and sprinkle with paprika.

Bake for 20 to 25 minutes.   *Makes 8 servings*

Broiled Tomatoes

Here is a simple procedure to add variety to luscious red tomatoes when you tire of serving them raw and sliced.

4 large ripe tomatoes
½ cup, or less, Cashonnaise (page 137) or Pimiento Cashew Cheese (page 135)

¼ cup whole-grain cracker crumbs, onion-flavored if possible
1½ teaspoons sweet basil

Wash and core tomatoes. Cut them in half horizontally.

Coat cut side of each tomato half with thin layer of Cashonnaise or

Pimiento Cashew Cheese, then sprinkle with cracker crumbs and sweet basil.

Broil tomatoes, cut side up, for 4 to 5 minutes or until tops are golden brown. *Makes 4 servings*

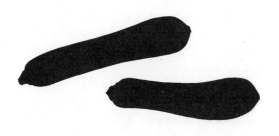

Summer Zucchini Boats

Many children don't like "mushy" zucchini. (Many grownups don't either!) These zucchini boats are crisp because they are broiled for only a few minutes, and the green onions and cheese sauce add flavor. To eat, pick them up and crunch!

6 small zucchini
½ cup chopped green
    onions
½ cup, or as needed,
    Pimiento Cashew
    Cheese (page 135)

Whole-grain cracker
    crumbs, onion-flavored
    if possible

Preheat broiler.

Wash zucchini and trim the ends; halve lengthwise. Sprinkle with chopped green onions and cover lightly with Pimiento Cashew Cheese; sprinkle with cracker crumbs.

Place boats on baking dish and broil until golden brown, watching closely so they do not get too dark. *Makes 6 servings*

Wonderful Spaghetti Sauce

Here is an exquisitely seasoned "healthful spaghetti sauce" that is good on any kind of pasta. It is also an important ingredient in the two recipes that follow.

2 tablespoons olive oil
1 small eggplant, chopped
1 small zucchini, chopped
1 green bell pepper,
    chopped
1 large onion, chopped
1 cup sliced mushrooms
1 clove fresh garlic,
    minced, or ½ teaspoon
    garlic powder

¼ cup water
1 jar (32 ounces) natural
    spaghetti sauce
2 teaspoons sweet basil
1 teaspoon sage
1 teaspoon salt
½ teaspoon dried oregano
½ teaspoon dried thyme
½ teaspoon ground cumin

Heat olive oil in large saucepan to point of fragrance. Add eggplant, zucchini, bell pepper, onion, mushrooms, and water, and cook over medium-low heat, stirring occasionally, for 5 to 10 minutes or until crisp-tender.

Add remaining ingredients. Simmer over low heat for 7 minutes, stirring occasionally.

Serves 8 to 10 when used as a sauce for pasta

Veggie Spaghetti Marzetti

This popular casserole can be used as an entrée or a side dish.

1 recipe Wonderful
    Spaghetti Sauce (recipe
    above)
1 package (8 ounces)
    Jerusalem artichoke
    spaghetti or other
    whole-grain spaghetti,
    cooked

1 cup chopped leeks or
    green onions
1 cup sliced pitted black
    olives
1 cup shredded soy
    mozzarella
2 teaspoons Italian
    seasoning

Preheat oven to 350°F.

Combine Wonderful Spaghetti Sauce and cooked spaghetti in large bowl, tossing thoroughly. Place mixture in 13 x 9-inch baking dish. Add single layers of leeks or green onions, olives, and shredded soy mozzarella. Sprinkle generously with Italian seasoning.

Bake for 20 to 25 minutes or until bubbly.

Makes 10 to 12 servings

Ratatouille à la Potato

A wonderfully nutritious meal that needs only a platter of raw carrots and celery to complete it.

1 recipe Wonderful
  Spaghetti Sauce (page
  85), made with only 2
  cups natural spaghetti
  sauce
2 large tomatoes, chopped
4 large potatoes, freshly
  baked

1 cup shredded soy
  mozzarella
1 cup chopped green
  onions
2 teaspoons Italian
  seasoning
  Vege-Sal to sprinkle

Heat Wonderful Spaghetti Sauce over medium heat, add chopped tomatoes, and simmer for 2 to 3 minutes.

Cut open hot baked potatoes. Generously spoon sauce into potatoes (sauce will spill down sides). Top with shredded soy mozzarella and green onions and sprinkle with Italian seasoning and Vege-Sal. Put potatoes in 350°F oven to melt cheese, if desired. Serve immediately.

Makes 4 servings

Good Shepherd's Pie

This old-fashioned vegetable pot pie with a Southern cashew twist makes a terrific entrée.

2½ cups Southern-Style
   Gravy (page 141)
 1 package natural onion-
   soup mix
 1 teaspoon Bakon
   seasoning
 2 teaspoons sweet basil
 1 teaspoon Vege-Sal
 2 cups diced potatoes
 1 cup thinly sliced
   carrots

2 cups shredded green
  cabbage
1 cup chopped celery
½ cup chopped green bell
  pepper
½ cup chopped red bell
  pepper
½ cup chopped onion
  Flaky Pie Crust (page
  44)

Preheat oven to 400°F.

Heat gravy in a saucepan. Stir in onion soup mix, Bakon seasoning, sweet basil, and Vege-Sal and simmer for 5 minutes, stirring. Remove from heat.

Place a steamer basket in a large pot over an inch or two of boiling water. Add the potatoes and carrots, steam until crisp-tender, and remove from steamer basket. Add cabbage, celery, bell peppers, and onion to the steamer basket and steam for 3 to 4 minutes. Add vegetables to gravy and mix gently.

Roll out half the pastry and place in a 9-inch pie plate. Fill with the vegetable-gravy mixture. Roll out the remaining pastry, cover filling, and trim excess pastry. Crimp edges of pie to seal well and cut a few slits in the top crust to allow steam to vent.

Bake for 30 minutes, or until golden brown and bubbling.

Makes 8 to 10 servings

Avocado Astoria Salad

If you can find organically grown, unwaxed apples, leave them unpared, for the red peel will add to the beauty of this delectable salad. Unfortunately, in today's world we must take into account the prevalence of waxes and pesticides and peel fruit when necessary.

2 cups diced apples
½ cup chopped walnuts
½ cup cubed ripe avocado
½ cup raisins
½ cup seedless green
    grapes, halved
    (optional)

3 tablespoons Palm
    Springs Fruit Dressing
    (page 142)
2 to 3 tablespoons pine
    nuts

Lightly toss together all ingredients except pine nuts. Serve in individual dishes, topped with pine nuts.   *Makes 4 to 6 servings*

Cruiser of Island Delights

This is a good dish to bring to a potluck or buffet. Your hostess will appreciate the festive look the dark green pineapple leaves and mounds of colorful fruit give to her table.

It's important to choose a good, ripe pineapple. Look for one with a yellow-orange, not green, hue; the middle leaves should pull out easily, and the bottom should smell sweet.

1 large fresh pineapple	1 cup sliced fresh peaches
2 medium-size ripe	or sweet mango
bananas, sliced	½ cup chopped nuts
1 cup orange sections	2 cups Orange-Pineapple
1 cup seedless green	Sauce (page 41)
grapes, halved	

Halve pineapple lengthwise, leaving each half with leaves intact. Remove pineapple flesh with a sharp knife and spoon, core, and cut into chunks. Chill empty halves while assembling other ingredients.

Toss pineapple chunks with sliced fruit and nuts. Chill mixture until ready to serve.

To serve, scoop fruit mixture into pineapple halves. Top with Orange-Pineapple Sauce. Use any leftover fruit to replenish the shell, or save it to blend into fruit drinks or smoothies.

Makes 6 to 8 servings

Tahitian Holiday

As with all fruit recipes, the ingredients should be ripe and fresh. There's no point in making a fresh fruit salad or dessert with inferior fruit! Here the Tangy Sweet Lemon Sauce adds a piquant flavor to the sweet juicy fruit.

1 medium-size ripe	2 medium-size ripe
honeydew melon	bananas, sliced
2 cups fresh pineapple	½ cup toasted slivered
chunks	almonds
1 cup cubed sweet ripe	1 recipe Tangy Sweet
mango	Lemon Sauce (page 40)
1 cup cubed ripe papaya	

Wash and halve honeydew. Scoop out seeds and discard. Remove honeydew flesh by making balls with melon scoop or spoon, leaving shells intact. Add rest of ingredients to melon balls and toss lightly.

Fill honeydew shells with fruit mixture. Chill until ready to serve. Serve topped with Tangy Sweet Lemon Sauce.

Makes 8 to 10 servings

Cantaloupe Castles

This recipe may inspire you to try other combinations of simple fruits and juice, served in natural containers.

All of these fruit combinations benefit by being chilled for an hour or so, but remember that they lose their freshness when chilled too long. Bananas, especially, may start to brown after a while.

2 medium-size ripe cantaloupes	2 medium-size ripe bananas, sliced
1 cup sliced fresh peaches, nectarines, or mangoes	¼ cup unsweetened pineapple juice
1 cup seedless green grapes, halved	

Cut cantaloupes in half; scoop out seeds and discard.

Mix together remaining fruit with pineapple juice. Fill cantaloupe halves with fruit mixture and chill for approximately ½ hour before serving.

Makes 4 servings

Summer Fresh Fruit Compote

A mixture of fresh fruit is wonderful in itself; served with Piña Colada Fruit Cream, it is heavenly.

2 cups sliced fresh peaches	1 cup fresh pineapple chunks
1 cup sliced fresh strawberries	1 cup fresh blueberries

2 medium-size ripe
    bananas, sliced

2 cups Piña Colada Fruit
    Cream (page 39)

Toss fruit together in large bowl. Chill for at least 1 hour before serving.

Serve in sherbet glasses, topped with Piña Colada Fruit Cream.

Makes 6 to 8 servings

Fresh Rainbow Tapioca

Icy green grapes, deep red strawberries, and bright peaches form beautiful layers of color in these parfaits.

2½ cups unsweetened
    pineapple juice
¼ cup minute tapioca
¼ cup honey
1 cup unsweetened
    crushed pineapple,
    drained
2 medium-size ripe
    bananas, sliced
1 cup sliced fresh
    strawberries

1 cup sliced fresh
    peaches
1 cup seedless green
    grapes, halved
⅓ to ½ cup Sunrise
    Crunchy Granola
    (page 17) or other
    granola, preferably
    fruit-sweetened

Combine pineapple juice, tapioca, and honey in saucepan. Let sit for 5 minutes, then place over medium heat, stirring constantly until mixture thickens, about 5 to 10 minutes. Remove from heat and stir in crushed pineapple and bananas.

Layer tapioca mixture and fruit in parfait glasses in this order: place strawberries in bottom of parfait glass, add thin layer of tapioca mixture, then peaches, then another thin layer of tapioca, then grapes. Chill for 1 hour. Sprinkle with granola, about a tablespoon for each parfait.

Makes 6 to 8 servings

. WORKING THE . PROGRAM

When we start to emphasize raw or lightly cooked vegetables, we get into real Seventh-Day Adventist territory, and the heart of the eating program that gives us long lives, glowing health, and slender bodies. Increasing consumption of fresh fruit is rarely a problem. Fruits are portable, convenient, and sweet—and everyone has at least *one* favorite fruit! But vegetables are important, too. Let's take a realistic look at why it seems so difficult for many of us to enjoy our share of vegetables!

In part, it's habit. Most of us are used to thinking of a meal according to the type of meat it contains. Vegetables are often an afterthought, perhaps a little bowl of lettuce or a mound of frozen peas. When you begin to give vegetables more importance—sometimes centering a meal around an assortment of vegetables—it all becomes much easier.

It will help to devote more space in your refrigerator to fruits and vegetables. Stuffing all of them into one drawer marked "produce" is an invitation to forget about them. Try devoting two drawers and a shelf or two to them.

But if you fill your refrigerator with unusual vegetables that you don't known how to cook, they will end up limp and moldy anyway! It's best to begin with those you are familiar with—raw carrot sticks, steamed broccoli, and baked potatoes are just as wonderful and nutritious as are more exotic vegetables. From there you can branch out, perhaps learning to cook a new vegetable every week.

Some people hate washing vegetables. One experienced cook told me it is much more pleasant when you wash them with warm water. As for peeling and chopping—unfortunately, these chores can't be eliminated entirely. Some people find the slicing and shredding disks on a food processor invaluable in helping with the cutting chores.

We have recommended several appliances that make healthful cooking easier—but a little, inexpensive collapsible metal steamer may become your favorite kitchen utensil of all. Steaming—the best cooking method for retaining nutrients—is quite easy once you get used to it, and a light steaming is the best way to preserve fresh flavors. Put about an inch of water in the bottom of a pan with a lid (the water should not touch the bottom of the steamer when it is placed in the pan) and bring it to a boil. Drop in the steamer with its vegetables, tightly cover the pan, and turn the heat down to medium. (To maintain steam pressure, be sure that the water continues to boil.)

Now comes the frustrating part. How long do you cook the vegetables? Cookbooks are vague on this question. The reason for the vagueness is that the length of cooking time depends on the kind of vegetable, its age, the size of the pieces—and the cook's preference for crisp, crisp-tender, or very tender texture. Some experimentation must be involved in this process. Just be careful not to burn yourself. Open the lid away from you and be sure you do not steam your fingers!

Table 8 provides approximate cooking times to help you judge when you should begin checking your steaming vegetables. When a recipe says "crisp-tender," it means the vegetable should be *just tender enough* to cut easily with a fork. The more health-conscious you are, the more you will want to eat your vegetables slightly on the raw side—but by all means, cook them the way you like them!

Table 8 • *Steaming Time in Minutes for Vegetables*

Artichokes, Jerusalem	25	Kohlrabi	10–20
Artichokes, small	15–20	Mustard greens	15
Asparagus tips	12	Okra, sliced	5
Beans, green	10	Okra, whole	15
Beans, lima, shelled	25–35	Parsnips, sliced	10–15
Beets, medium	20	Peas, green, shelled	5
Broccoli	10	Peppers, green or red	10
Brussels sprouts	15	Potatoes, sweet, sliced	25–30
Cabbage, green or red	15	Potatoes, white, sliced	25–30
Carrots, sliced	15	Pumpkin, in chunks	35–40
Carrots, whole	30	Rutabagas, sliced	20–30
Cauliflower	15	Spinach	7–10
Celery, sliced	10–20	Squash, summer, sliced	5
Celery root, sliced	35	Squash, winter, in	
Chard	10	chunks	25
Collards	30	Tomatoes, sliced	5
Corn, fresh	5–7	Turnip greens	25–30
Eggplant, sliced	10	Turnips, sliced	15–20
Kale	20–25		

Another difficult question is, What do you put on cooked vegetables? For those concerned about weight and/or cholesterol, butter is out. We have a friend who simply loves a plateful of steamed vegetables seasoned with herbs and a little salt. If this is a description of your own taste, indulge yourself! But most of us want something more. Ellen White herself recommended making vegetables palatable with sweet fresh cream. But that was 150 years ago, when cows were healthier and pesticide residues had not become concentrated in their milk—and when people got much more exercise through their work, which made the ingestion of cholesterol less dangerous than it is for most of us today. Ellen White foretold of the day when we would have to be very careful about our consumption of dairy products, and for many people this has become a real concern. While the plan in this book does not dictate a drastic elimination of all dairy products, you will notice that none of the recipes here contain any dairy products, which will make it easier for those who wish to cut back.

Some people like cooked vegetables sprinkled with nutritional yeast. If you are not concerned about weight loss, a little soy margarine may be just the thing. Many people love a tablespoon of Pimiento Cashew Cheese (page 135) on cooked green vegetables, and Southern Style Gravy (page 141) or avocado and herbs on baked potatoes. You will probably find there are some vegetables you will enjoy completely without added fat. A good, moist sweet potato requires nothing at all—sometimes it seems more like a dessert than a vegetable! Some find vegetables such as Brussels sprouts and spinach delectable with only a little salt and perhaps a sprinkling of onion powder and lemon juice.

The following chart can help you decide how to season fresh vegetables. Choose one of the herbs listed to go with the vegetable, or use a combination of two or more. A pinch of each will suffice (a "pinch" is usually a quarter to a half a teaspoon); be more generous with fresh herbs, if you have access to them. Add a little salt (unless you are on a salt-restricted diet) and some fresh lemon juice. The flavor of the lemon juice makes it possible to cut back on the amount of salt. There are also several good vegetable-based seasonings on the market that contain little or no salt.

For many vegetables, a combination of onion, bell pepper, and garlic is the most delicious flavor-enhancer. You may choose to add these ingredients in powder form (even bell pepper comes finely ground, found in the herb section) to cooked vegetables, or you may add them fresh, chopped, directly to the steamer basket.

Most people who think they don't like certain vegetables such as cabbage, broccoli, or cauliflower find that they enjoy them when they are stir-fried in a wok Chinese-style and served over rice.

Herbal Seasoning Combinations for Vegetables

Beans, dried: Sweet basil, oregano, dill, savory, sage, coriander, cumin, garlic, parsley, bay leaf, onion–garlic–bell pepper combination

Beans, green: Sweet basil, dill, marjoram, rosemary, thyme, oregano, savory, onion–garlic–bell pepper combination

Beans, lima: Sweet basil, chives, marjoram, savory, onion–garlic–bell pepper combination

Beets: Tarragon, dill, sweet basil, thyme, bay leaf, cardamon seed

Broccoli: Tarragon, marjoram, oregano, sweet basil, "cheese" sauce (recipes for several "cheese" sauces are found in Chapter 4, pages 135–140)

Brussels sprouts: Sweet basil, dill, savory, caraway, thyme

Cabbage: Caraway, celery seed, savory, tarragon, dill, Bakon seasoning, onion–garlic–bell pepper combination

Carrots: Sweet basil, dill, marjoram, thyme, parsley, coriander

Cauliflower: Sweet basil, rosemary, savory, dill, tarragon, "cheese" sauce

Cucumbers: Tarragon, sweet basil, savory

Eggplant: Sweet basil, thyme, oregano, rosemary, sage, "cheese" sauce, onion–garlic–bell pepper combination

Fruit salad: Mint, rosemary, lemon balm, coriander

Green salads, dressings for: Sweet basil, parsley, chives, tarragon, lemon thyme, dill, marjoram, oregano, rosemary, savory, mint

Onions: Oregano, thyme, sweet basil

Peas: Sweet basil, mint, savory, oregano, dill, onion–garlic–bell pepper combination

Potatoes: Dill, chives, sweet basil, marjoram, savory, parsley, "cheese" sauce, onion–garlic–bell pepper combination

Spinach: Tarragon, thyme, oregano, rosemary

Squash: Sweet basil, dill, oregano, savory, Italian seasoning, onion–garlic–bell pepper combination

Tomatoes: Sweet basil, oregano, dill, garlic, savory, parsley, bay leaf

In addition to the use of herbs, cooks of natural foods often combine simple foods that complement one another. As Frankie Lappe pointed out in *Diet for a Small Planet,* when you begin with fresh, natural, high-quality ingredients, almost any combination can work. It's fun to use what you already have on hand in devising new combinations. Here are some ideas for pleasing vegetable combinations that are common in Adventist circles:

Bok choy and celery cabbage

Corn and pimientos

Cauliflower and green peas

Pearl onions, mushrooms, and green peas

Carrot slices and green lima beans

Mushrooms and green peas

Diced carrots in nest of French-style green beans

Tomatoes, onions, and zucchini

Green lima beans in acorn squash halves

Acorn squash rings with green peas

Carrots, cabbage, and celery

Celery and mushrooms

Okra, onions, and tomatoes

Carrots and green peas

Brussels sprouts and celery

Summer squash, tomatoes, and onions

Green lima beans and corn

Green cabbage, onions, and green bell pepper

Brussels sprouts and carrot slices

Broccoli and cauliflower florets

Corn and green peas

Eggplant, zucchini, onions, and tomatoes

In addition to these ideas, there are many vegetable-based casseroles in this chapter and entrées in Chapter 4 that are absolutely delicious. The vegetables used in an entrée or casserole may be "counted" as part of your vegetable intake for the day.

For those who aspire to the peak of health: Eat at least one raw vegetable per day, or a raw vegetable salad. A platter of raw vegetables is sometimes the easiest thing to serve; it doesn't always require even salad dressing. And it may be the only way your child will eat vegetables—raw and plain!

Some people believe they don't like vegetables because they have only been acquainted with the canned or frozen variety, or "fresh" ones long past their prime. You may be stunned when you discover the difference in produce that is fresh, picked at the peak of ripeness, and free from decay. This is why it is beneficial to patronize good roadside stands and farmer's markets, and to center your meals around fruits and vegetables that are in season. Especially if you are de-emphasizing meat in your diet, you will want to spend a little extra time hunting down the finest produce. Where do you find this extra time? Buy quantities of dried beans and grains and the other foods that don't spoil quickly, and spend your shopping time on the more fragile foods.

If you want to, you can grow your own sprouts! This means you can do your organic gardening in your kitchen, especially nice in winter when greens are expensive and not abundant. Simply take a glass quart jar and put in it 3 tablespoons of seeds (alfalfa seeds are good to begin) and some water (at least enough to cover the seeds) and fasten a mesh screen or piece of cheesecloth over the top of the jar with a rubber band. Leave it in a dark place overnight. The next morning invert the jar, draining the water through the mesh. Add fresh water and rinse, then drain again. Then place the jar on its side, or inverted in a bowl—once again in a dark place. Repeat the rinsing and draining process two times a day, or three times a day in summer. In a few days the sprouts should be long enough (one to two inches long). Place the jar in the sun for a few hours to "green up" the sprouts, then use them as needed in sandwiches, salads, baked potatoes, and recipes.

• S U M M A R Y •

1. The risk of developing chronic degenerative diseases drops dramatically when fruits and vegetables are increased so that they make up 50 percent of the diet. Americans currently consume an average of only 8.6 percent of their calories as fruits and vegetables.

2. Liberal use of fruits and vegetables in your diet may allow you to

eat as much as you want to without gaining weight. The fiber in these foods and in legumes and whole grains makes it possible to lose weight without counting calories.

3. Fiber also helps to reduce the buildup of cholesterol, thus decreasing your risk of a heart attack. The best sources of this fiber are apples, beans, and oats.

• This Week's Guide to Success •

Increase your fruit and vegetable intake to 5 servings per day.
Even better would be 6 or more servings per day.

Spend most of your market time with the "greengrocer."
Don't skimp on fruits and vegetables—they are your best allies in the fight for health and slimness.

Keep your meals simple.
Vary your diet from meal to meal, but don't eat too many kinds of foods at one time.

When selecting your fruits and vegetables for the day, choose colorfully!

Enjoy your food and eat all you need to maintain energy and health.
But please do not overeat.

4

· *Principle No. 4* ·

Go Low on Fat

*Both the blood and the fat of animals are
consumed as a luxury. But . . . these should not
be eaten. Why? Because their use would make a
diseased current of blood in the human system.*
—*Ellen G. White*

Chris writes:
A few years ago my family faced a major crisis. All waited
anxiously for what seemed like an eternity in the hospital waiting
room as my father underwent bypass surgery. He had long been
plagued with atherosclerotic disease, and now not only his heart but
both legs were in danger because of the disease's effect on his circulation.

At last the family was told that he would have to lose a leg. I will
never forget what he said when I was finally able to see him: "Christine, I never thought I would lose my leg because of the way I lived.
I just never thought . . ."

Strangely, I was reminded of a humorous poem that tells the story
of a town with a problem. The town is located near a precipice, and
its citizens continually fall off the edge of the cliff and injure themselves. The town council meets to determine how to remedy the situation. One faction demands the purchase of an ambulance to be
kept at all times at the bottom of the cliff, ready to take the victims
immediately to the hospital. The other group of townspeople suggests
that a fence be built at the edge of the cliff, so that no one will fall off
in the first place!

When it comes to health, unfortunately, a lot of us have been "ambulance people." Most people wait until they become the victims of
chronic degenerative disease before doing anything about it.

Philosopher Charles Pierre Peguy once said, "When a man dies, he
dies not of a disease, but of his entire life."

99

The solution to our escalating problems with chronic degenerative disease lies in building the fence of "life-style management"—learning to take control of our lives so we may live *happily, healthily ever after!*

My father decided to get busy with the "construction work" of building a fence. He had lost a leg to the poor circulation that resulted from his atherosclerosis; he did not want to lose his life. He began to follow dietary principles similar to the ones outlined in this book, including eliminating cholesterol and saturated animal fat from his diet; he began an exercise program as soon as it was possible. His high blood pressure and cholesterol levels are now under control, and he has dropped forty-five unwanted pounds. By the way, he's a strapping six-foot three-inch gentleman, handsome, healthy, and happy as ever.

Would you like some help in building a fence against obesity, heart disease, and other chronic degenerative diseases? This chapter will provide you with some of the materials!

First, let's take a look at what should be called the nation's *real* "Big Mac Attack": coronary heart disease. Heart attacks occur every twenty-five seconds in the United States and kill every sixty seconds. They are the most common cause of death in the United States. According to the American Heart Association, the mortality rate from coronary heart disease due to atherosclerosis is 700,000 lives per year.

Atherosclerosis is the condition in which fat and cholesterol are deposited on the vulnerable inside walls of the blood vessels. This formation, known as plaque, slowly narrows the blood vessels, diminishing the blood flow. Severe clogging of the arteries causes the heart to cry out in pain (angina pectoris). Ultimately, as plaque formations create obstructions in the arteries, a heart attack occurs.

The picture is really very serious. Some researchers have indicated that as much as 75 percent of all American men aged twenty-two to forty-five have coronary atherosclerosis. And 65 percent of American women have cholesterol levels that place them in the high-risk category. Dr. Tazewell Banks, director of the Heart Station at Washington, D.C.'s, General Hospital, states that "46 percent of all American men at age twenty-two already have the beginnings of coronary heart disease." Further, researchers at Louisiana State University, determined recently that out of thirty-five *youths* who died between the ages of seven and twenty-four, *all but six* had early signs of atherosclerosis. When diseases such as this one begin to show up in our youth, it is definitely time to take a serious look at what we can do to prevent them.

At the heart of the matter are our dietary practices! While McDonald's is serving 140 hamburgers per second around the world and 45.8 million Americans still eat at fast-food restaurants daily, the National Institutes of Health (NIH) and other organizations are making some strong statements about America's eating habits. The NIH and other agencies are urging a dramatic cutback in dietary fat. The Center for Science in the Public Interest (CSPI) indicates that the average American consumes 89 grams of fat a day.

Some fast-food meals contain 60 or more grams of fat! According to the CSPI, a regular order of fries can contain 11.5 grams of fat; a chocolate shake, 9 grams; and the "Big Mac Attack," 34 grams. A Double Whopper with Cheese at Burger King has a fat whopping 61 grams of fat just by itself. (Is that why it's called a Double Whopper?)

What if you don't frequent fast-food outlets? Well, let's take a look at what's placed on the kitchen table in many American homes:

Table 9 • *Saturated Fatty Acids in Selected Foods*

Food	Saturated Fatty Acids	
	% of Fat	Grams
MEAT, POULTRY, FISH		
Beef, cooked, 3 oz.	50	8
Hamburger	47	8
Round	46	6
Steak, sirloin	48	13
Roast, rib	47	16
Veal	54	6
Lamb chop, with bone, 4.8 oz.	55	18
Pork chop, with bone, 3.5 oz.	38	8
Ham, 3 oz.	39	7
Chicken, fryer, 3 oz.	32	2–3
Hen, 3 oz.	34	7
Fish sticks, 3.2 oz.	25	2
Salmon, 3 oz.	20	1
DAIRY PRODUCTS AND EGGS		
Milk, whole, 1 cup	56	5
2%, 1 cup	56	3
Canned, evaporated, 1 T.	56	0.7
Cheese, cheddar, 1 oz.	56	5
Cottage, creamed ¼ cup	56	1.5
Cream, 1 oz.	56	5

Food	Saturated Fatty Acids	
	% of Fat	Grams
Cream, half-and-half, 1 T.	56	1
Whipping, heavy, 1 T.	56	3
Ice cream, ½ cup	56	4
Egg, large	33	2
NUTS AND SEEDS		
Nuts, almonds, 1 oz. (not roasted)	8	1
Cashews, 1 oz. (roasted)	17	2
Peanuts, 1 oz. (roasted)	22	3
Peanut butter, 1 T.	25	2
Walnuts, 1 oz.	5	1
Sunflower seeds, 1 oz.	13	2
FATS AND OILS		
Butter, 1 T.	56	6.5
Lard, 1 T.	38	5
Margarine, soft, 1 T.	18	2
Oils, corn, 1 T.	10	1.4
Olive, 1 T.	11	1.5
Soybean, 1 T.	15	2
Peanut, 1 T.	18	2.5
Cottonseed, 1 T.	25	3.5
Mayonnaise, 1 T.	18	2
Salad dressings, 1 T.	13	1
DESSERTS AND SWEETS		
Cake, 1 piece	33	1–3
Candy, 1 oz.	27	3
Chocolate-covered peanuts	25	3
Fudge, plain	50	2
Cookies, 1 average	33	1
Danish pastry, 4¼-in. diameter	33	5
Ice cream, ½ cup	56	4
Pudding, average, 1 cup	50	5
MISCELLANEOUS		
Avocado, ½ medium	19	3.5
Macaroni and cheese, 1 cup	45	10
Pizza with cheese, 2½ oz.	33	2
Pancake	50	1
Waffle, 7-in. diameter	29	2
Soup, cream, 1 cup	30	3–4
Soybeans, cooked, ½ cup	20	1

Table 10 • *Sources of Fat in the U.S. Diet*

Food Group	% of Total Fat
Meat (including poultry and fish)	34.2
Cooking and salad oils	14.5
Shortening	13.2
Dairy products (excluding butter)	12.9
Margarine	7.2
Legumes and cocoa	5.0
Butter	3.1
Eggs	3.0
Lard (direct use)	2.7
Other edible fats and oils	1.9
Grain products	1.4
Fruits and vegetables	0.9
	100.0

U.S. Department of Agriculture, *Fats and Oils Situation,* May 1980, p. 21

Take a mean look at meat, even the so-called lean meats. Even when the obvious fat is carefully trimmed away, the hidden fat that remains still makes up 30 to 50 percent of the meat.

It's important to note that cholesterol is found *only in animal products* (meat and dairy products), as is the highest percentage of saturated fats. Seventy percent of the saturated fat consumed by Americans comes from animal products.

Our bodies need cholesterol to process fat—but we don't need *one milligram* of cholesterol from our food. Our own bodies manufacture ample cholesterol to do the job—four times as much as the average American gets from his daily diet. The cholesterol in food has been exposed to the air; it has oxidized and formed toxic substances, unlike the pure cholesterol made in the body. Studies have shown that it is this oxidized cholesterol that may damage the arteries. When we consume additional amounts of cholesterol, we simply create a dangerous surplus. Also, the typical high-fat diet is generally deficient in fiber, which, among other things, serves as a vehicle to remove excess bile acids and cholesterol from the body. If these bile acids and cholesterol are not removed, they create a greater risk for colon cancer. And the deadly duo of fat and cholesterol contributes to the formation of plaque on the inside walls of the blood vessels.

Table 11 · *Cholesterol in Foods*

Food	Mg Cholesterol in 3½ oz. (100 g)
HIGH	
Brains	2000
Egg yolk, fresh	1500
Egg, whole	550
Kidney, uncooked	375
Caviar or fish roe	300
Liver	300
Butter	250
Sweetbreads (thymus)	250
Oysters	200
Lobster	200
Heart, uncooked	150
Crabmeat	125
Shrimp	125
Cheese, cream	120
MEDIUM	
Cheese, cheddar	100
Lard or other animal fat	95
Veal	90
Whipping cream	85
Cheese (25–30% fat)	85
Beef, uncooked	70
Fish, steak	70
Fish, fillet	70
Lamb, cooked	70
Pork	70
Cheese spread	65
Margarine (⅔ animal, ⅓ vegetable)	65
Mutton, flesh only, uncooked	65
Chicken, flesh only	60
Ice cream	45
Sour cream	45
LOW	
Cottage cheese, creamed	15
Milk, fluid whole	22
Milk, fluid skim	3
Egg white	0
Fruits	0
Nuts	0

Food	Mg Cholesterol in 3½ oz. (100 g)
Grains	0
Vegetables	0

Compiled and calculated from USDA Handbook No. 8

The 1984 National Institutes of Health Consensus Conference asked this question: "Does the deposit of dietary cholesterol and saturated fat really make any difference in the development of atherosclerosis?" The consensus was: Yes, it can make a difference, a difference that can have fatal consequences.

In an early Seventh-Day Adventist book on nutrition and health compiled in 1897, this statement is found: "Both the blood and the fat of animals are consumed as a luxury. But . . . these should not be eaten. Why? Because their use would make a diseased current of blood in the human system." Although written in 1896 by the remarkable Ellen G. White, we hear the echoes of these words in the scientific statements of our day. What early Adventists termed "a diseased current of blood," we now call atherosclerosis.

Adventists are one of the most highly studied groups in the world. Since the 1950s, scientists in the United States, Japan, Australia, Poland, Norway, New Zealand, the Netherlands, and the Caribbean Islands have published over 200 scientific papers on studies involving tens of thousands of Adventists. Scientists have been intrigued by the connection between the life-style of this group and their greater longevity, particularly their much lower rates of death due to chronic degenerative disease.

A major study involving more than 25,000 Adventist adults over a period of twenty years indicated that a vegetarian Seventh-Day Adventist life-style can indeed lead to longer life. Dr. David Snowdon, an assistant professor of epidemiology at the University of Minnesota, and Dr. Roland L. Phillips, a professor of epidemiology at Loma Linda University, suggest that an Adventist woman aged twenty-five has an average of sixty-three more years to live, while a non-Adventist woman the same age will average fifty-four more years. The data suggest that vegetarian Adventist men aged twenty-five will enjoy fifty-nine more years of life in comparison to non-Adventist men, who will average only forty-seven more years. It appears that the earlier one embraces the complete Adventist life-style, the greater quality of life and longevity one can expect.

Tables 12 and 13 show the impact of the Seventh-Day Adventist life-style on mortality rates due to various diseases in comparison with those of the general population.

The results of one significant study are shown in Table 13, which compares the death rates of various groups of Adventist men. These groups had very similar life-styles, differing mainly in the amount of animal fat included in their diets. Those who followed closely the dietary program of the Adventist church (the total vegetarians) had only 12 percent of the expected mortality rate from coronary heart disease!

A vegetarian diet can substantially lower the serum cholesterol level. In a 1978 study, Seventh-Day Adventist lacto-ovo vegetarians (vegetarians who include milk and eggs in their diets) were found to have lower serum cholesterol levels than the general United States population. However, vegetarian Adventists who excluded *all* animal products from their diets, even milk and eggs, were found to have the *lowest* levels. Another study reported in the September 1984 *American Journal of Clinical Nutrition* found lacto-ovo vegetarians to have lower levels of cholesterol in their blood. Referring to this research, an article in the January 1985 *Journal of the American Dietetic Association* stated: "Results suggest that differences seen in the levels of various lipids and lipoproteins between nonvegetarians and people adopting a vegetarian lifestyle are due to differences in diet."

The effectiveness of dietary changes in lowering blood cholesterol should not be underestimated! Because of the way Chris's family cooks and eats, her entire family enjoys the advantages of low blood cholesterol levels. Her husband's cholesterol level is 120, while her own level and those of her two teenagers and her ten-year-old are all under 100!

These levels are not unusual among vegetarians. In third-world nations, where most people do not have access to or cannot afford our highly fatty foods, cholesterol levels are often under 100.

In view of the fact that over 63 million Americans are plagued with some form of heart disease (a staggering one person in four!), sweeping measures should be taken to halt the onslaught of this most devastating disease.

Some who already have atherosclerosis may be wondering if there is help for them. Can diet help clear the arteries of the damage already done?

The data from a number of regression studies done around the

Table 12 • *Death Rate of Seventh-Day Adventists Due to Various Causes Compared with the General Population*

*Adventist
Death Rate*

*Death Rate in General
Population = 100%*

Coronary heart disease—55%

Stroke—53%

Cirrhosis of the liver—13%

Diabetes—55%

Peptic ulcer—42%

Suicide—31%

Lung cancer—20%

Emphysema—32%

All cancer—59%

All causes—59%

Table 13 • *Coronary Death Rate for Adventist Men with Various Dietary Habits Compared with the General Population*

*Adventist
Death Rate*

*Death Rate in General
Population = 100%*

14%—Total vegetarian

39%—Vegetarian plus milk and eggs

56%—Meat included in diet

37%—Nonvegetarian

12%—Vegetarian

R. L. Phillips et al., *Journal of Clinical Nutrition,* vol. 31: S191–S198, 1978.

globe suggest that the impossible may be possible. Atherosclerosis can be reversed! Researchers from the University of Southern California School of Medicine demonstrated that lowering blood cholesterol through low-fat diet and cholesterol-lowering drugs can effect dramatic changes in atherosclerotic arteries. Dr. David H. Blankenhorn, chief investigator of the study, stated: "This study demonstrates that we now have the wherewithal to turn heart disease around in its early stages."

Japanese scientists reported that on a diet containing no meat, no cheeses, and no butter and limited amounts of milk and eggs, they were able to halt and even to reverse atherosclerosis in 167 people. In other research worldwide, the data coming in suggest that a vegetarian diet can decrease vessel blockage. In the Netherlands, researchers reported that individuals on a lacto-ovo vegetarian diet with no more than 100 milligrams of cholesterol per day were able to arrest or reverse atherosclerosis over a two-year period. Dr. Dean Ornish of the University of California, San Francisco, recently demonstrated that with diet and exercise alone—without the use of drugs—patients were able to reverse their atherosclerosis and begin to open up clogged arteries. In each case this was accomplished during one year on a program of good diet and exercise. All of these studies showed that heart disease can be reversed with a diet that is *low* in saturated fats and cholesterol and high in whole plant foods. In fact, if you use only recipes similar to those described in this book, your cholesterol intake will be almost nil!

Some people mistakenly believe that a vegetarian diet is nutritionally unbalanced or inadequate. But studies on lacto-ovo vegetarians and total vegetarians have indicated that these groups receive adequate intakes of all nutrients. In fact, the average intake of food approximates or surpasses the amounts recommended by the National Research Council's Food and Nutrition Board. The only "deficiency," if you call it that, was in weight. Vegetarians generally weigh less than the average person.

With respect to the most stubborn myths about the inadequacy of a vegetarian diet, namely deficiencies of B_{12}, protein, and iron, we offer this statement from a position paper on vegetarian eating by the American Dietetic Association:

> The American Dietetic Association affirms that a well-planned diet, consisting of a variety of largely unrefined plant foods supplemented with some milk and eggs (lacto-ovo vegetarian diet)

meets all known nutrient needs. Furthermore, a total plant diet can be made adequate by careful planning, giving proper attention to specific nutrients which may be in a less available form or in lower concentration or absent in plant foods.

The American Dietetic Association recognizes that a growing body of scientific evidence supports a positive relationship between the consumption of a plant-based diet and the prevention of certain diseases.

What's this? *Careful planning?* Maybe you're thinking that a vegetarian diet will be too much trouble if you have to plan that carefully!

But wait. The fact is, achieving health on a *meat-centered* diet requires *much more* careful planning than the planning required for a healthful plant-based diet. To extend your life when you eat meat you must be careful to keep your intake of cholesterol and saturated fat below certain recommended levels each day—not to mention current concerns over the prevalence of hormones, chemicals, and certain animal diseases. For most vegetarians, *careful planning* means *eating a wide variety of foods*—and this is something that *all* people, vegetarian or not, must strive for if they want to live healthy lives!

It was once thought that to obtain all essential amino acids, one needed to combine two different plant foods. But current research shows that there is actually no need for this. The combining of foods to ensure adequate amino acid balance is important only for infants in some underdeveloped countries. There is no food containing protein (with the exception of gelatin) that does not have all the essential amino acids.

Adequate protein is easily obtained if one consumes enough calories to maintain body weight. If one-third of these calories are from beans and greens, another third from potatoes and grains, and another third from fruit, 13 percent of one's calories would be protein (the Food and Nutrition Board's recommended allowance of protein is 10 percent of total calories consumed; the minimum allowance is 5 percent of total calories). If this diet was nutritionally diluted so that 50 percent of the calories came from sugar and oil, the diet would still be 6½ percent protein, and would still meet the minimum requirement. In other words, when one eats enough calories to maintain proper body weight, it is very difficult to produce a protein deficiency.

What about maintaining adequate levels of vitamin B_{12} on a vegetarian diet? *Nutrition Reviews* makes this statement:

> In man, the small intestines as well as the colon contain microflora which synthesize significant amounts of vitamin B_{12}. People subsisting on vegetarian diets depend on this source as well as ingested microorganisms for their vitamin B_{12} nutriture.

We follow vegetarian diets that contain a wide variety of nutritious foods, and both of us feel comfortable that our B_{12} needs are being met. But because this issue is still controversial in some circles, and because we would hate to see people avoiding a healthy vegetarian (or near-vegetarian) way of life simply out of fear of a B_{12} deficiency, we see nothing wrong with taking a B_{12} supplement, as many scientific groups recommend.

Seventh-Day Adventists advocate a vegetarian life-style for a longer, healthier, more satisfying life. But while the typical high-fat American diet is clearly an invitation to trouble, you may not be ready to make the transition to a completely vegetarian diet. However, by following the Menu Planner and beginning to substitute vegetarian entrées for meat, you will benefit step by step. The more you do, the more you will realize your goals of weight and cholesterol reduction.

Following is a selection of recipes for vegetarian entrées that are high in fiber and low in fat. In place of high-fat foods such as salad dressings, mayonnaise, gravies, and cheeses, they offer some delicious alternatives that are nutritious and heart saving.

Are you ready to build your fence? Here are the materials to help you.

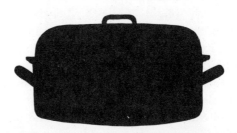

· R E C I P E S ·

Cooking Beans

Some people don't realize that the protein food group in-
cludes legumes, nuts, and seeds in addition to meat and meat
products. Seventh-Day Adventists rely on legumes as a major
source of protein. These nutrient-rich, high-fiber foods pro-
vide good biological protein without the high-fat drawbacks
of meat. Adventist cooking combines legumes, whole grains,
fresh vegetables, and herbs in a variety of ways to create the
most savory and aromatic of low-fat entrées.

Here are some techniques that will enable you to cook
dried beans so that they turn out perfectly every time—and
that will help you avoid what is euphemistically called the
"distress" that can come from eating them!

The Old-Fashioned Method

Consult Table 14 below to determine the correct amounts of beans
and water. Place the beans in a large colander and pick them over to
remove all particles of grit, dirt, or sand and any damaged beans.
Rinse well, rubbing beans between palms to clean them thoroughly.

Table 14

Beans (1 cup dry measure)	Water	Cooking Time	Yield
Baby limas	2 cups	1½ hours	1¼ cups
Black beans	4 cups	2 hours	2½ cups
Black-eyed peas	3½ cups	1½ hours	2½ cups
Garbanzos	4 cups	5 hours	2½ cups
Great Northern beans	4 cups	2 hours	2½ cups
Kidney beans	4 cups	2½ hours	2½ cups
Lentils & split peas	3 cups	1¼ hours	2¼ cups
Pinto beans	4 cups	2½ hours	2 cups

Beans (1 cup dry measure)	Water	Cooking Time	Yield
Red beans	4 cups	3 hours	2 cups
Small white beans (navy, etc.)	4 cups	2 hours	2½ cups
Soybeans	4 cups	5 hours	2 cups

Cover beans with water and let soak several hours or overnight.

Drain soaked beans and place in a heavy pot with a tight-fitting lid. Cover with the required amount of water and cook slowly until done, as indicated. If needed, add more water. Add salt (1 teaspoon for each cup of dry beans) near end of cooking time (if you add it sooner, it will toughen the skins of the beans and slow cooking).

Many people stay away from beans because they cause flatus or gas. The guilty substances in beans are two starches (stachyose and raffinose) that are not broken down by the starch-digesting enzyme that is normally present in the digestive tract. Instead, the two starches remain in the tract, where they come into contact with certain bacteria that break them down into carbon dioxide and hydrogen, the two main components of gastrointestinal "gas." One method to help alleviate the problem is to add 2 tablespoons of whole fennel seed to the cooking water before cooking the beans. Another method is as follows:

1. In the morning: Wash beans and place in heavy pot. Cover with amount of water needed for cooking. Let soak all day.

2. In the evening: Place beans and water in freezer. Freezing helps break up starch molecules mentioned above.

3. When ready to cook: Heat beans in water, which has become ice. When melted, add meat tenderizer that contains papain. Cook for required time in this same water. The tenderizer contains salt, so you need not add more. (Papain is an enzyme derived from papaya that breaks down the troublesome starches. Indo brand meat tenderizer is free of harmful additives and is available at most health food stores. Adolph's Meat Tenderizer also contains papain and is available at most supermarkets in a variety that does not contain MSG. An alternative is to cook the beans with six crushed papain enzyme tablets, available at local health food stores. The tablets contain no salt, so it will be necessary to salt beans toward the end of the cooking time.)

The Pressure Cooker Method

One way to cut down on the time involved in preparing beans is to cook the soaked beans and seasonings (including salt) in a pressure cooker. Follow the manufacturer's directions; it usually takes less than 30 minutes.

The Crockpot Method

This is the easiest method of all, and makes bean cookery a snap if you're daunted by all that soaking, freezing, simmering, etc. Jan admits that she would not dream of cooking beans any other way! It's easy to dump beans in the pot with a bunch of seasonings and vegetables, turn on the pot, and forget about it until the savory smells coming from the kitchen remind you that you have a potful of beans cooking themselves.

More good news is that cooking beans in the crockpot seems also to alleviate the problem of bean-related "distress."

Carefully sort and wash beans and place in crockpot. Add water to cover beans by 2 to 3 inches as indicated. Add salt, seasonings, and vegetables. A teaspoonful of either honey or a good olive oil added to the pot will further enhance the flavor of the beans.

Cook on high setting overnight or number of hours indicated in Table 15. If the mixture gets too thick, stir in a little water toward end of cooking time.

The Meatless Roast

Perhaps you're a meat-and-potato person. Beans on the dinner plate are fine, but "where's the beef?" You may want to try a meatless dish that looks something like a meat loaf. Adventist cooks are famous for their vegetarian roasts. You can become famous, too—at least in your own home—with this guide to creating your own roast, vegetarian style.

Table 16 will allow you to be inventive when preparing a roast, or simply to use the ingredients you happen to have on hand. Please don't forget to include the oil and salt.

Table 15 •

Legumes (1 pound)	Water	Salt	Seasonings
Red beans (pinto, kidney, or red beans)	Cover 2–3 in. above beans	2 tsp.	2 tsp. sweet basil 1 tsp. ground coriander 1 tsp. Bakon seasoning 1 tsp. ground cumin 1 tsp. sage ½ tsp. garlic powder 1 tsp. olive oil
White beans (Great Northern, navy)	Cover 2–3 in. above beans	2 tsp.	2 tsp. sweet basil 1 tsp. ground coriander 1 tsp. Bakon seasoning 1 pkg. onion soup mix 1 bay leaf ½ tsp. garlic powder 1 tsp. olive oil
Black beans	Cover 2–3 in. above beans	2 tsp.	2 tsp. sweet basil 1 tsp. ground coriander 1 tsp. Bakon seasoning 1 tsp. ground cumin ½ tsp. garlic powder 2 T. lemon juice* 1 tsp. olive oil
Black-eyed peas	Cover 2 in. above beans	2 tsp.	2 tsp. sweet basil 1 tsp. ground coriander 1 tsp. Bakon seasoning 2 bay leaves 1 package onion soup mix ½ tsp. garlic powder 1 tsp. olive oil
Lentils	Cover 2 in. above lentils	1½ tsp.	1 tsp. sweet basil ½ tsp. sage ¼ tsp. thyme ½ tsp. garlic powder 2 T. lemon juice* 1 tsp. olive oil
Split peas	Cover 2 in. above peas	1½ tsp.	1 tsp. sweet basil 1 tsp. sage 1 tsp. Bakon seasoning ½ tsp. garlic powder ¼ tsp. thyme 2 T. lemon juice* 1 tsp. olive oil

* Stir fresh lemon juice into legumes *just before serving.*

Crockpot Beans

Vegetables	Cooking Time	Yield
1 bun. green onions, chopped 1 green bell pepper, chopped 1 cup chopped tomatoes or 1 cup tomato sauce	7–8 hrs. on high	5 to 6 cups
1 bun. chopped green onions 1 cup chopped celery	6–7 hrs. on high	5 to 6 cups
1 bun. green onions, chopped 1 green bell pepper, chopped	7 hrs. on high	5 to 6 cups
1 bun. green onions, chopped 1 cup chopped celery	6 hrs. on high	5 to 6 cups
1 onion, chopped 1 bell pepper, chopped 1 cup chopped tomatoes	5 hrs. on high	5 to 6 cups
1 bun. green onions, chopped 1 cup chopped celery ½ cup chopped green bell pepper ½ cup chopped red bell pepper	5 hrs. on high	5 to 6 cups

Table 16 • *Guide to Creating*

Protein (1 cup)	Whole Grain (2 cups)	Chopped Nuts (½ cup)	Liquid (1 to 1½ cups)
Pinto beans	Brown rice (cooked)	Almonds	Soy milk
Kidney beans	Rolled oats (uncooked)	Pecans	Nut milk (cashew, almond)
Garbanzo beans	Whole-grain bread crumbs (dry)	Cashews	Tomato sauce
Lentils	Whole-grain cereal flakes	Walnuts	Pimiento Cashew Cheese (page 000) (1 cup)
Tofu	Whole-grain cracker crumbs	Peanuts	Broth from cooked vegetables
Soy cheese (shredded)	Grape-Nuts	Sunflower seeds	Mushroom soup (from natural mix)

You may serve a meatless roast with gravy over steamed brown rice or mashed potatoes—or serve with a simple accompaniment of steamed vegetables and a tossed salad. Leftover roast may be refrigerated and sliced for sandwiches.

Preheat oven to 350°F.

In a large bowl combine one ingredient from each of the first five columns of the chart (protein, whole grain, chopped nuts, liquid, and binding). Add three ingredients from the Chopped Vegetables column and two Seasonings (1 teaspoon of each), 2 tablespoons oil, and 1 teaspoon salt. Mix well.

Press mixture into an oiled 9 x 5-inch loaf pan. Bake for 45 minutes. **Makes 6 to 8 servings**

Your Own Meatless Roast

Binding	Chopped Vegetables (Any three)	Seasonings (Any two)	All Roasts
3 T. peanut butter	1 red or green bell pepper, chopped	1 tsp. coriander	
2 T. soy flour	1 onion, chopped or 1 cup chopped green onions	½ tsp. sage	
½ cup cooked cereal (oatmeal, Bearmush, millet, etc.)	1 cup chopped celery	½ tsp. oregano	1½ tsp. salt 3 T. oil
3 T. tapioca	1 cup chopped tomatoes	1 tsp. Bakon seasoning	
3 T. potato flour	½ cup chopped black olives	1 tsp. sweet basil	
½ to 1 cup mashed potatoes	3 cloves minced garlic	1 tsp. Italian seasoning	

Haystacks

A Haystack is one of the successful complete meals that Adventists have devised in their quest to develop simple, natural, flavorful meals. They are popular in Adventist circles everywhere. Jan loves them because they're quick and easy—and because her children love them!

Precise amounts are not given for the ingredients, for they will depend on the number and appetites of the eaters, and on their preferences. Try ½ cup of chips per serving, ½ cup of beans, a couple of tablespoons of Pimiento Cashew Cheese, and ¼ to ½ cup of each of the remaining ingredients—or whatever you think would taste best. Top with Guacamole!

This meal is also excellent when a baked potato or cooked brown rice is substituted for the mound of corn chips.

Whole-grain corn chips
Cooked pinto beans (see
    table, page 111)
Pimiento Cashew Cheese
    (page 135)
Onions, diced, or green
    onions, chopped
Tomatoes, diced

Green leaf lettuce,
    shredded
Fresh spinach, chopped
Black olives, sliced
Guacamole (page 139)

Mound chips on plate; scoop beans on top of chips; spread Pimiento Cashew Cheese over beans. Add remaining ingredients in layers. Top with guacamole.

Macaroni and Cheese Casserole

This lovely dish may be served as a side dish or an entrée. Try it with Jerusalem artichoke macaroni and don't even mention that this dish is a healthy one! Everyone will love this alternative to the classic macaroni and cheese, which is loaded with fat and cholesterol.

If you don't have soy cheese on hand, just leave it out—the casserole will still be delicious.

1 package (8 ounces)
    whole-grain macaroni
1 cup frozen green peas
1 cup sliced mushrooms
1 bunch green onions,
    chopped
2 to 2½ cups Pimiento
    Cashew Cheese (page
    135)
1 teaspoon dried sweet
    basil

1 teaspoon ground
    coriander
1 teaspoon Bakon
    seasoning (optional)
½ teaspoon salt
1 cup shredded soy
    cheddar
    Paprika

Prepare macaroni according to package directions, but cook only until barely tender.

Preheat oven to 350°F.

Drain macaroni and place in large bowl. Add remaining ingredients except for soy cheddar and paprika; mix well. Pour into 11½ x 8-inch baking dish and top with soy cheddar. Sprinkle with paprika. Bake for 20 to 25 minutes. **_Makes 6 to 8 servings_**

Mexican Mountains

Chris's family eats dinner for breakfast (they don't like doing dishes in the evening!) This is a hearty meal that Chris makes convenient by placing the potatoes in a cold oven the night before. She sets her alarm for an hour before she would normally get up; she makes her way to the kitchen and turns on the oven; then she goes back to bed! When the alarm goes off the second time, the potatoes are done and ready to be "layered."

Use fairly generous amounts of each topping—¼ to ½ cup of each. Remember, these are called mountains!

Medium-large baking potatoes

Cooked pinto beans (see table, page 111)

Tomatoes, chopped

Black olives, pitted and sliced

Green onions or leeks, chopped

Pimiento Cashew Cheese (page 135)

Crushed corn chips

Prepare baked potatoes: Preheat oven to 375°F. Scrub and pierce potatoes and bake for 1 to 1¼ hours.

Turn oven down to 350°F. Cut open potatoes and layer with desired amounts of following ingredients in order given: pinto beans, tomatoes, olives, and green onions. Top with a layer of Pimiento Cashew Cheese and crushed corn chips. Bake for 12 minutes.

Baked Vegetable Rotini

Rotini are little spiral or corkscrew-shaped noodles. If you can't find them at first, you may substitute spaghetti, broken in half before cooking.

This dish may serve as an entrée or side dish, and is delicious the next day, served cold as a pasta salad.

1 package (8 ounces) Jerusalem artichoke rotini

1 green bell pepper, cored, seeded, and chopped

1 red bell pepper, cored, seeded, and chopped

1 bunch green onions, chopped

1 cup sliced pitted black olives, chopped

1 cup chopped zucchini

1 cup sliced mushrooms

1 cup chopped tomatoes

1½ teaspoons dried sweet basil

1 teaspoon ground coriander

1 teaspoon Vege-Sal or ½ teaspoon salt

1 teaspoon Bakon seasoning (optional)

1 recipe Pimiento Cashew Cheese (page 135)

1 cup shredded soy mozzarella

1 teaspoon Italian seasoning

Prepare rotini according to package directions, but cook only until barely tender.

Preheat oven to 350°F.

Drain rotini and place in large bowl. Add bell peppers, green onions, olives, zucchini, mushrooms, and tomatoes, and stir.

Stir sweet basil, coriander, Vege-Sal or salt, and optional Bakon seasoning into Pimiento Cashew Cheese. Add this mixture to bowl of rotini and vegetables and stir in gently but thoroughly. Pour into 13 x 9-inch baking dish and top with soy mozzarella and Italian seasoning.

Bake for 20 minutes or until bubbly.   *Makes 10 to 12 servings*

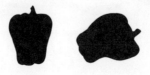

Pesto Sauce

This sauce adds wonderful flavor to the following two recipes. Use it to flavor other Italian dishes, even plain cooked pasta.

½ cup pine nuts or pecans
¼ cup olive oil
⅓ cup water
¼ cup fresh lemon juice

½ cup fresh or dried sweet
    basil leaves
3 cloves garlic
½ teaspoon salt

Place all ingredients in blender and blend until smooth.

Makes approximately 1½ cups

Pesto Tofu Manicotti

The flavor of this dish is remarkably good. You may use any kind of large pasta that is suitable for stuffing.

1 package (8 ounces)
    whole-grain manicotti
    shells (or other large
    stuffing shells)
1 pound tofu
1 teaspoon onion salt
1 bunch green onions,
    chopped
1 green bell pepper, cored,
    seeded, and chopped

1 cup sliced mushrooms
1 recipe Pesto Sauce
    (recipe above)
1 jar (32 ounces) natural
    spaghetti sauce
2 cups shredded soy
    mozzarella
    Italian seasoning

Cook manicotti shells according to package directions.
Preheat oven to 350°F.

Place tofu cake in large bowl and mash with fork, adding onion salt (texture should be similar to cottage cheese). Add green onions, bell pepper, mushrooms, and Pesto Sauce and mix well.

Drain manicotti shells and stuff with pesto-tofu mixture. Place side by side in 13 x 9-inch baking dish. Cover with spaghetti sauce. Top with soy mozzarella and sprinkle liberally with Italian seasoning.

Bake for 25 minutes or until bubbly.

Makes 12 servings

Pesto! Pesto! Pie

The Pesto Sauce is so good that we had to include another recipe that contains it. Pungent flavor in a flaky crust is impossible to resist! This recipe has become a specialty with Jan and a favorite with her friends.

1 recipe Flaky Pie Crust (page 44)	1 small zucchini, thinly sliced
½ pound tofu	1 cup chopped green onions
½ teaspoon onion salt	
½ recipe Pesto Sauce (page 121)	½ cup sliced mushrooms
1½ cups shredded soy mozzarella	½ cup chopped green bell pepper
	Italian seasoning
½ to ¾ cup natural spaghetti sauce	

Preheat oven to 400°F.

Roll out half of pie crust dough and line 9-inch pie plate. (Save other half of dough in refrigerator or freezer to use in another recipe.) Crimp edges, then prick sides and bottom of crust to prevent puffing. Bake for 10 minutes. Set aside.

Make filling: Turn oven down to 350°F. Place tofu cake in large bowl and mash with fork, adding onion salt (texture should be similar to cottage cheese). Add Pesto Sauce and ½ cup shredded soy mozzarella and mix well.

Spread spaghetti sauce in bottom of baked pie shell; add a layer of zucchini, then green onions, then pesto mixture, mushrooms, and green bell pepper. Top with remaining soy mozzarella. Sprinkle generously with Italian seasoning.

Bake for 20 to 25 minutes. ***Makes 6 to 8 servings***

Oat Pecan Burgers

We like to make a batch of these burgers every week or so to freeze and use as needed. They are good served cold in sandwiches as well as in the recipes which follow.

These have a better flavor than most vegetarian burgers

and a much better texture. When Chris was demonstrating how to make them for a television cooking show, the cameraman demanded that she give him the recipe! If you want to make a smaller amount, cut the recipe in half.

4 cups water	2 teaspoons onion powder
½ cup soy sauce	1 teaspoon Bakon
⅓ cup canola oil	seasoning
1 cup chopped pecans or	1 teaspoon ground
walnuts	coriander
¼ cup nutritional yeast	1 teaspoon dried sage
flakes	4 cups rolled oats
2 teaspoons garlic powder	
1 tablespoon dried sweet	
basil	

Place all ingredients except rolled oats in a large pan, stir well, and bring to a slow boil over medium-low heat. Stir in rolled oats and immediately remove from heat. Cover and set aside to cool.

Preheat oven to 350°F.

Form oat mixture into 3-inch patties and place on oiled baking sheets. Bake for 15 minutes on each side.

Makes approximately 20 burgers

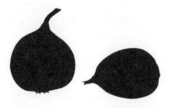

Ratatouille Noodle Casserole

If you have Oat Pecan Burgers on hand, this dish is easy to put together. (In fact, if you don't have any burgers on hand and don't feel like making any, it's also good without them!) It's another good example of the Adventist practice of using combinations of vegetables for flavor and health, often in casseroles that are baked only "until bubbly"—not until all the flavor and nutrition is cooked out of the vegetables!

1 package (8 ounces) whole-grain noodles
1 small green bell pepper, cored, seeded, and cut into thin strips
1 small red bell pepper, cored, seeded, and cut into thin strips
½ large onion, sliced into thin strips
1 small zucchini, cut into thin strips
½ cup thin strips of eggplant
1 jar (32 ounces) natural spaghetti sauce
1 cup water
2 teaspoons dried sweet basil
1 teaspoon ground coriander
1 teaspoon Vege-Sal or ½ teaspoon salt
1 teaspoon Bakon seasoning
6 Oat Pecan Burgers (recipe above), cut into strips
½ to 1 cup shredded soy cheddar
Italian seasoning

Prepare noodles according to package directions, but cook only until barely tender.

Preheat oven to 350°F.

Drain noodles and pour into 13 x 9-inch baking dish. Place bell peppers, onion, zucchini, eggplant, spaghetti sauce, water, basil, coriander, Vege-Sal or salt, and Bakon seasoning in large bowl and stir until blended. Gently stir in Oat Pecan Burger strips. Spread mixture over noodles.

Top with shredded soy cheddar and sprinkle with Italian seasoning.

Bake for 15 minutes or until bubbly.   *Makes 10 servings*

Burger Stroganoff

Another hearty meal that is strong on flavor.

1 package (8 ounces) whole-grain flat noodles
1 recipe Southern-Style Gravy (page 141)
1 package natural onion-soup mix
1 cup sliced mushrooms
1 small green bell pepper, cored, seeded, and thinly sliced
½ large onion, cored, sliced, and thinly sliced
4 Oat Pecan Burgers, cut into strips

Prepare noodles according to package directions, but cook only until barely tender.

Preheat oven to 350°F.

Prepare Southern-Style Gravy, adding package of onion soup mix after it has thickened. Simmer 1 minute, then stir in mushrooms, bell pepper, and onion, and simmer over low temperature for 5 minutes, stirring occasionally.

Drain noodles and pour into 11½ x 8-inch baking dish. Place Oat Pecan Burger strips on noodles.

Pour vegetable-gravy mixture over burgers and noodles. Bake for 12 to 15 minutes or until bubbly. **Makes 8 to 10 servings**

California Sunshine Burgers

Vegetarian cooks take pride in not serving up a pale imitation of nonvegetarian food. After all, vegetarian food is real food! However, sometimes it's comforting to make a dish such as this one, with familiar all-American appeal.

This is an easy recipe to divide or multiply to serve one or a crowd.

2 whole-grain hamburger buns, halved
2 tablespoons low-calorie mayonnaise or Cashonnaise (page 137)
4 Oat Pecan Burgers (page 122), baked

4 thick tomato slices
1 cup Pimiento Cashew Cheese (page 135)
Sliced pitted black olives
Chopped green onions

Preheat oven to 350°F.

Place hamburger bun halves in baking dish. Spread bun halves with low-calorie mayonnaise or Cashonnaise. Top each half with an Oat Pecan Burger and a thick slice of tomato. Drizzle generously with Pimiento Cashew Cheese. Top each burger with a few sliced black olives.

Bake for 12 to 15 minutes. Garnish with chopped green onions. Serve hot. **Makes 4 servings**

Oat-Pecan Steaks
Over Mashed Potatoes

6 medium boiling potatoes
   Vege-Sal or salt
1 recipe Southern-Style
   Gravy or
   Creamy Oat-Mushroom
   Gravy
1 small onion, sliced into
   thin strips

½ medium green bell
   pepper, cored, seeded,
   and sliced into thin
   strips
6 Oat-Pecan Burgers (page
   122), baked

Boil potatoes and mash with Vege-Sal or salt to taste.

Bring gravy to a simmer, add onion and bell pepper, and simmer over low heat for 5 to 7 minutes.

Mound hot mashed potatoes on plates, top each mound with a burger, and spoon gravy generously over each serving.

Makes 6 servings

Deep-Dish Pizza Pie

An easy and delicious variation of this dish is Pizza Hoagies. Instead of the pie crust, use whole-wheat hoagie buns (also known as hero or submarine buns). Cut them in half and layer with Oat Pecan Burgers and other ingredients as described below. Bake or broil in the oven till cheese is melted.

1 recipe Flaky Pie Crust
   (page 44)
6 Oat Pecan Burgers
   (page 122), crumbled
1½ cups natural spaghetti
   sauce or pizza sauce
1 cup sliced mushrooms
1 cup chopped tomatoes
1 cup Pimiento Cashew
   Cheese (page 135)

1 green bell pepper,
   cored, seeded, and
   chopped
1 bunch green onions,
   chopped
1 cup sliced pitted black
   olives
1½ cups shredded soy
   mozzarella cheese
   Italian seasoning

Preheat oven to 400°F. Press Flaky Pie Crust dough into 13 x 9-baking dish, and prick, on bottom and sides, to avoid puffing. Bake for 10 to 12 minutes.

Turn oven down to 350°F.

Place layers of following ingredients in baked pie shell, in order given: crumbled burgers, spaghetti sauce, mushrooms, tomatoes, Pimiento Cashew Cheese, bell pepper, green onions, olives, and shredded soy mozzarella. Sprinkle generously with Italian seasoning.

Bake for 25 to 30 minutes. Remove from oven and let stand for 10 minutes before serving. **Makes 10 to 12 servings**

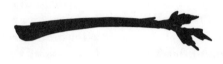

Out-of-This-World Lentil Stew

Those who love lentils will love this stew. It may also be made in the crockpot; add water to a level 2 inches above the lentils and cook for 5 hours on high.

1 pound dried lentils
½ cup raw brown rice
1 cup chopped carrots
1 cup chopped celery
1 cup chopped green bell pepper
1 onion, chopped
2 tomatoes, chopped
1 cup natural tomato sauce
1 tablespoon molasses
1½ teaspoons salt
1 teaspoon dried sweet basil
½ teaspoon dried sage
½ teaspoon dried thyme
¼ teaspoon garlic powder
Juice of ½ lemon

Wash and sort lentils. Place in large pot, cover with water by 2 to 3 inches, bring to boil, and cover. Turn down heat and simmer for 30 minutes. Add brown rice and simmer for 30 minutes. Add remaining ingredients except for lemon juice and simmer for another 15 minutes.

Add lemon juice just before serving. **Makes 8 to 10 servings**

Empañadas

Don't pass over this festive Latin-inspired recipe—it's well worth the effort. All you need to accompany it is a tossed salad and perhaps some Nature's Best Baked Corn (page 78).

2 tablespoons olive oil
1 cup chopped green
  onions
1 cup sliced mushrooms
½ cup chopped green bell
  pepper
½ cup chopped red bell
  pepper
2 cloves garlic, minced
4 Oat Pecan Burgers (page
  122), crumbled
½ cup sliced pitted ripe
  olives
½ cup cooked brown rice

1 teaspoon dried sweet
  basil
2 teaspoons Bakon
  seasoning
1 teaspoon ground
  coriander
1 teaspoon ground cumin
½ teaspoon ground sage
1 teaspoon Vege-Sal or ½
  teaspoon salt
½ cup tomato sauce
1 recipe Flaky Pie Crust
  (page 44)

Preheat oven to 400°F.

Heat olive oil in skillet over medium heat; add green onions, mushrooms, bell peppers, and garlic. Sauté for 5 to 10 minutes, stirring occasionally. Add crumbled burgers and rest of ingredients except for Flaky Pie Crust and mix well.

Roll out pie crust dough thinly between sheets of plastic wrap and cut into 4-inch circles. You should have about 1½ dozen.

Place about 2 tablespoons burger mixture on each circle of pastry. Fold pastry over and seal edges with a fork, gently shaping into a half moon.

Transfer empañadas to a baking sheet and bake for 20 minutes or until golden brown.   *Makes about 1½ dozen*

Spinach Lasagna

1 package (8 ounces) whole-grain lasagna noodles
2 tablespoons olive oil
2 cups chopped onion
2 cups sliced mushrooms
1 cup chopped green bell pepper
2 cloves garlic, minced
2 cups chopped tomatoes
1 bunch fresh spinach, washed, drained, and chopped
1 cup chopped celery
1 jar (32 ounces) natural spaghetti sauce

2 teaspoons dried sweet basil
1 teaspoon dried sage
1 teaspoon Bakon seasoning
¼ teaspoon dried thyme
½ teaspoon dried oregano
¼ teaspoon dried marjoram
Salt to taste
3 cups shredded soy mozzarella
2 teaspoons Italian seasoning

Prepare lasagna noodles according to package directions.

Preheat oven to 350°F.

Heat olive oil in large saucepan over medium heat; add onions, mushrooms, bell pepper, and garlic. Sauté for 3 to 4 minutes, stirring occasionally. Add rest of ingredients, except soy mozzarella and Italian seasoning, and simmer over low heat for 10 minutes, stirring occasionally.

Lightly oil 13 x 9-inch baking dish. Layer half the cooked lasagna noodles in bottom of dish, then add layers of half the spinach-tomato sauce and 1½ cups soy mozzarella, and sprinkle with 1 teaspoon Italian seasoning. Make a second layer of cooked noodles, then layer on rest of spinach-tomato sauce with remaining 1½ cups soy mozzarella, and sprinkle with remaining 1 teaspoon Italian seasoning.

Bake for 25 minutes or until bubbly. ***Makes 12 servings***

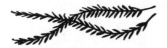

Savory Stuffed Peppers

1 cup raw brown rice
1 package natural onion-
   soup mix
5 large, whole green bell
   peppers
1 tablespoon olive oil
½ cup chopped green bell
   pepper
½ cup chopped red bell
   pepper
½ cup sliced mushrooms
2 cloves garlic, minced
½ cup chopped raw
   cashews, well rinsed

2 to 3 tablespoons soy
   sauce
1 teaspoon ground
   coriander
1 teaspoon dried sweet
   basil
½ teaspoon dried oregano
½ teaspoon dried sage
½ cup Pimiento Cashew
   Cheese (page 135)
1 to 2 tablespoons whole-
   grain cracker crumbs,
   onion-flavored if
   possible

Preheat oven to 350°F.

Cook brown rice according to package directions, adding onion-soup mix to cooking water. Stir occasionally while cooking (it may be necessary to add a little more water).

Wash whole green bell peppers, cut off the tops, core, and remove seeds.

Heat oil in large skillet over medium-high heat; add chopped bell peppers, mushrooms, garlic, cashews, soy sauce, coriander, sweet basil, oregano, and sage. Sauté for 5 minutes or until vegetables are tender, stirring occasionally. Remove from heat and add 2 cups cooked brown rice and ½ cup of the Pimiento Cashew Cheese. Mix well.

Stuff peppers with vegetable mixture. Top each with thin layer of remaining Pimiento Cashew Cheese and sprinkle with cracker crumbs.

Bake for 25 minutes or until peppers are tender.

Makes 5 servings

Nutty Brown Rice Roast

1 cup raw brown rice
1 package natural onion-
   soup mix
3 tablespoons olive oil
1 cup chopped green
   onions
1 green bell pepper,
   cored, seeded, and
   chopped
2 cloves garlic, minced
2 tablespoons soy sauce
1 cup soy milk
1 cup mashed tofu
2 cups whole-grain cracker
   crumbs

1 cup chopped cashews,
   well rinsed
¼ cup natural peanut
   butter
2 teaspoons dried sweet
   basil
1 teaspoon ground
   coriander
1 teaspoon Bakon
   seasoning
½ teaspoon dried sage
2 cups Southern-Style
   Gravy (page 141)

Cook brown rice according to package directions, adding onion-soup mix to cooking water. Stir occasionally while cooking (it may be necessary to add a little more water).

Heat olive oil in skillet over medium heat, add green onions, bell pepper, and garlic. Sauté approximately 5 minutes, stirring occasionally. Stir in soy sauce and remove from heat.

Combine cooked brown rice with sautéed vegetables and rest of ingredients, except gravy. Mix well. Spoon into lightly oiled 11½ x 8-inch baking dish.

Bake for 35 to 40 minutes. Serve with Southern-Style Gravy.

Makes 6 to 8 servings

Almond Brown Rice Croquettes

Serve these with Southern-Style Gravy (page 141) or Creamy Oat-Mushroom Gravy (page 141) as an entrée.

1 cup raw brown rice
1 package natural onion-
    soup mix
2 cups whole-grain cracker
    crumbs, onion-flavored
    if possible
1 cup crumbled tofu
½ cup sliced mushrooms
1 cup prepared natural
    mushroom soup
1 bunch green onions,
    chopped

½ cup sliced almonds
¼ cup chopped parsley
¼ cup almond butter
2 tablespoons olive oil
1 teaspoon dried sage
1 teaspoon dried sweet
    basil
1 teaspoon ground
    coriander
1 teaspoon salt

Preheat oven to 350°F.

Cook brown rice according to package directions, adding onion-soup mix to cooking water. Stir occasionally while cooking (it may be necessary to add a little more water).

Combine cooked rice with 1 cup of the cracker crumbs and all remaining ingredients in large bowl. Form into 12 croquettes or patties, roll in remaining cracker crumbs to coat, and place on lightly oiled baking dish.

Bake for 15 minutes on each side or until golden.

Makes about 12 croquettes

Burrito Pie

Chris served this dish when one of her daughter's friends was visiting. The friend turned to Chris's daughter and said seriously: "You don't know how lucky you are!"

4 to 6 whole-wheat tortillas
2 to 3 cups cooked pinto,
    kidney, or red beans
    (see table, pages 111–
    112)

1 cup chopped tomatoes
1 cup chopped green
    onions
1 cup sliced pitted black
    olives

1 to 1½ cups Pimiento Cashew Cheese (page 135)	1 cup shredded soy cheddar or mozzarella Paprika

Preheat oven to 350°F.

Layer half of ingredients in 11½ x 8-inch baking dish, in this order: tortillas, beans, tomatoes, green onions, olives, and a thin layer of Pimiento Cashew Cheese. Repeat layers. Top with shredded soy cheese and sprinkle with paprika.

Bake for 20 minutes or until bubbly.   ***Makes 8 to 10 servings***

Black Bean Olé

Adventist cookery has an affinity for Mexican cookery— beans, rice, raw vegetables, and "cheese," which make for a very nutritious meal with a south-of-the-border flavor. Here are two festive recipes that will quickly become favorites. Serve with Guacamole (page 139)!

3 cups cooked brown rice	1 bunch green onions, chopped
3 cups cooked black beans, on the soupy side (see table, page 111)	1½ cups Pimiento Cashew Cheese (page 135)
2 cups chopped tomatoes	2 cups crushed whole-grain corn chips
1½ cups fresh corn kernels	
1½ cups sliced pitted black olives	

Preheat oven to 350°F.

Layer ingredients in a 13 x 9-inch baking dish, in order given.

Bake for 20 minutes or until bubbly.   ***Makes 10 to 12 servings***

Enchiladas

Sauce:

3 cups natural tomato sauce

1½ cups chopped green onions

½ cup chopped green bell pepper

1 cup chopped tomato

1 cup sliced pitted ripe olives

1 teaspoon garlic powder

1 teaspoon ground cumin

1 teaspoon sweet basil

1 teaspoon ground coriander

1 teaspoon Bakon seasoning

½ teaspoon salt

Filling:

1 tablespoon olive oil

1 cup chopped green onions

1 cup chopped green bell pepper

4 cups crumbled cooked Oat Pecan Burgers (page 122)

1 teaspoon Bakon seasoning

1 teaspoon sweet basil

1 teaspoon ground cumin

1 teaspoon ground coriander

1 tablespoon soy sauce

12 corn tortillas

1 cup shredded soy cheddar

1 cup shredded soy mozzarella cheese

Preheat oven to 350°F.

Make the sauce: Bring the tomato sauce to a simmer in a saucepan. Add the remaining sauce ingredients and simmer for approximately 8 minutes, stirring occasionally. Keep warm.

Make the filling: Heat the olive oil in a skillet, add the green onions and bell peppers and sauté until tender, about 2–3 minutes. Add the crumbled burgers and the seasonings and stir well. Set aside.

Dip each tortilla in the sauce, top with a couple of spoonfuls of filling, and roll up. Place the enchiladas in a lightly oiled 13 x 9-inch baking dish. Cover with remaining sauce and sprinkle with the grated cheese.

Bake for 20 minutes or until bubbly. *Makes 6 to 8 servings*

Bean Sandwich Spread

What do you serve on sandwiches if you've decided to give up the old tuna standby? Here is a delicious alternative. Try it stuffed into pita pockets, with sprouts, sliced avocados, and chopped tomatoes.

4 cups cooked beans, mashed	½ cup chopped green onions
1 cup chopped celery	1 teaspoon salt
⅔ cup Cashonnaise (page 137)	½ teaspoon onion powder
	½ teaspoon garlic powder

Combine all ingredients well.　　*Makes approximately 6 cups*

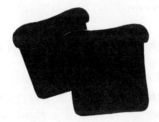

Pimiento Cashew Cheese

At last—the famous Pimiento Cashew Cheese. This is Chris's version of an Adventist standard. It's simple to make and adds flavor to all kinds of recipes. It can also be used as a dip for raw vegetables or a delicious salad dressing. We serve it to our kids with raw zucchini and broccoli and cauliflower florets to get them to eat raw vegetables.

As always, be sure to use nutritional yeast flakes (not powder). Also, please use fresh lemons. (Most people prefer the sharp flavor of a full ¼ cup of lemon juice in this sauce, especially if it's to be used in casseroles. If it's a little too strong for you, reduce the quantity.)

If the mixture stalls while blending, turn off the blender, add a little more water, and try again. (You will need to use a little more water anyway to make a thinner sauce for use in recipes where it is "drizzled.")

1 cup water
1 cup raw cashews, well
   rinsed
1 jar (4 ounces)
   pimientos, undrained
¼ cup nutritional yeast
   flakes
¼ cup fresh lemon juice
   (juice of 2 lemons)

2 tablespoons unhulled
   sesame seeds
1½ teaspoons onion
   powder
1 teaspoon salt
½ teaspoon garlic powder
1 teaspoon Bakon
   seasoning (optional)

Place all ingredients in blender and blend until creamy smooth, approximately 4 minutes.

Store in the refrigerator in tightly sealed plastic containers or glass jars. It will keep for about 10 days.

Makes 2½ to 3 cups

Sunflower Pimiento Cheese

This cheese sauce is not quite as creamy as one made with cashews, but we include it for two very important reasons. Sunflower seeds are less expensive than cashews; and those who are allergic to nuts may substitute this sauce for Pimiento Cashew Cheese. Moreover, it has a subtly different flavor that many will enjoy.

1 cup raw sunflower seeds
1¼ cups water
1 jar (4 ounces)
   pimientos, undrained
¼ cup nutritional yeast
   flakes
¼ cup fresh lemon juice
   (juice of 2 lemons)
2 tablespoons unhulled
   sesame seeds

1½ teaspoons onion
   powder
1 teaspoon salt
½ teaspoon dried sweet
   basil
½ teaspoon garlic powder
1 teaspoon Bakon
   seasoning (optional)

Place sunflower seeds and water in blender and blend 3 to 4 minutes, until smooth. Add remaining ingredients and blend until smooth. (You may need to add a little water.)

Makes approximately 3 cups

Cashonnaise

This is a wonderful substitute for mayonnaise, creamy and delicious! One tablespoon of traditional mayonnaise contains almost a tablespoon of fatty empty calories. However, one tablespoon of Cashonnaise has only a little over a teaspoon of cashews, which are not empty calorie foods but a source of protein, vitamins, and minerals.

Most mayonnaise substitutes become runny after sitting in the refrigerator for a few days. This "mayonnaise" retains enough body to help bind potato salads and pasta salads and to use as a spread that won't make sandwiches soggy.

What gives it texture is not egg yolks (those natural sources of calories and cholesterol!), but kosher gelatin. (For information on how to order Emes kosher gelatin, see page 204.) If you wish, you may substitute 1 teaspoon regular unflavored gelatin for the 1½ teaspoons kosher gelatin called for in the recipe.

1½ teaspoons unflavored kosher gelatin
¼ cup cool water
1 cup raw cashews, well rinsed
1 tablespoon nutritional yeast flakes
2 teaspoons honey
1½ teaspoons onion powder

1½ teaspoons salt
½ teaspoon dried sweet basil
½ teaspoon ground coriander
½ teaspoon garlic powder
1 cup boiling water
¼ cup fresh lemon juice (juice of 2 lemons)

Place gelatin in blender with cool water. Let soak while preparing other ingredients.

To blender add rest of ingredients except boiling water and lemon juice. Place lid on blender with insert removed; turn on blender and immediately begin to pour boiling water in steady stream through opening in lid. After all water has been added, continue to blend until very creamy, approximately 3 to 4 minutes. No cashew pieces should be visible! Finally, briefly blend in lemon juice.

Pour into jar with tight-fitting lid. Refrigerate several hours until set. (Stored in the refrigerator, this and the other "mayonnaise" recipes will keep for 10 days or more.)

Makes approximately 2½ cups

Tahinionnaise

Instead of spreadable fat, how about some spreadable nutrition? Because tahini is made from sesame seeds, this "mayonnaise" may be used by those who can't tolerate nuts. A word of warning: Though many enjoy the flavor of tahini, it may be a bit strong for those who are not used to "health foods." These people might do better to try the recipe that follows.

You may substitute 1 teaspoon regular unflavored gelatin for the kosher gelatin.

2 teaspoons unflavored
   kosher gelatin
¼ cup cool water
1 cup tahini (sesame seed
   butter)
1 tablespoon nutritional
   yeast flakes
2 teaspoons honey
1½ teaspoons onion
   powder

1½ teaspoons salt
1 teaspoon dried sweet
   basil
½ teaspoon ground
   coriander
½ teaspoon garlic powder
1 cup boiling water
¼ cup fresh lemon juice
   (juice of 2 lemons)

Place gelatin in blender with cool water. Let soak while preparing other ingredients.

To blender add rest of ingredients except boiling water and lemon juice. Place lid on blender with insert removed; turn on blender and immediately begin to pour boiling water in steady stream through opening in lid. After all water has been added, continue to blend until very creamy, approximately 3 to 4 minutes. Finally, briefly blend in lemon juice.

Pour into jar with lid. Refrigerate several hours, until set.

Makes approximately 2½ cups

Sunflower Seed Mayonnaise

1½ teaspoons unflavored
   kosher gelatin
¼ cup cool water
1 cup boiling water

1 cup raw sunflower seeds
1 tablespoon nutritional
   yeast flakes
2 teaspoons honey

1½ teaspoons onion
   powder
1½ teaspoons salt
½ teaspoon dried sweet
   basil
½ teaspoon garlic powder

1 teaspoon Bakon
   seasoning (optional)
1 cup boiling water
¼ cup fresh lemon juice
   (juice of 2 lemons)

Place gelatin in blender with cool water. Let soak for 10 minutes.

Add boiling water and blend briefly. Add rest of ingredients except lemon juice. Blend until very creamy, approximately 3 to 4 minutes. No sunflower pieces should be visible. Finally, briefly blend in lemon juice.

Pour into jar with a tight-fitting lid. Refrigerate several hours until set.   ***Makes approximately 2½ cups***

Hummus

As one taster said: "This is great! It tastes just like hummus!"

It is hummus, and makes a great dip for raw vegetables or bits of toasted pita, a spread for breads, or a salad dressing (add a little more garbanzo liquid or water when using as a dressing). One favored way to use it is to stuff pita bread with raw vegetables such as shredded red cabbage, alfalfa sprouts, shredded carrots, sliced olives, green onions, and chopped tomatoes—then drizzle generously with hummus. Eat with a fork (the brave may try their hands). Try any of your favorite raw vegetable combinations.

2 cups cooked garbanzo
   beans (canned will do)
⅓ cup garbanzo liquid or
   water
¼ cup tahini (sesame seed
   butter)

¼ cup fresh lemon juice
   (juice of 2 lemons)
4 cloves garlic, crushed
1 tablespoon olive oil
2 teaspoons onion powder
1 to 1½ teaspoons salt

Place all ingredients in blender and blend until smooth.

                  Makes approximately 2½ cups

Guacamole

In addition to serving on Haystacks (page 117), try Guacamole as a salad dressing, a sandwich spread (with alfalfa sprouts and tomatoes), a dip, an ingredient in stuffed pitas, or as a topping for Mexican-style dishes. A tip to remember: the dark, bumpy "alligator skin" avocados make the best guacamole.

There's nothing better!

2 ripe avocados, peeled and mashed with fork
1 tablespoon fresh lemon juice
1 teaspoon onion powder
¼ teaspoon garlic powder
½ teaspoon salt
¼ cup water
1 tomato, chopped (optional)
¼ cup chopped green onions

Place first six ingredients in blender and blend until smooth. Fold in chopped tomato and green onions. *Makes approximately 2 cups*

Sunflower Seed Sour Cream

Use this as a healthful alternate topping for baked potatoes.

¾ cup raw sunflower seeds
1½ cups water
½ cup Soyagen (soy protein powder)
2 teaspoons onion powder
1½ teaspoons salt
1 teaspoon dried sweet basil
½ teaspoon garlic powder
½ cup fresh lemon juice (juice of 4 lemons)

In blender place sunflower seeds and water and blend until smooth, approximately 3 to 4 minutes. Add rest of ingredients except lemon juice and continue to blend until creamy.

Fold in lemon juice with spatula or spoon. Pour into jar, cover, and chill. *Makes approximately 3 cups*

Southern-Style Gravy

This gravy is perfect for mashed potatoes—or try over whole-grain noodles. Its pale color is attractive to some (definitely southern style!), but if you prefer darker gravy, you may add a few drops of Kitchen Bouquet.

With some blenders it may be best to add the warm water gradually through the lid, as with the mayonnaise recipes.

2 cups warm water	2 teaspoons onion powder
½ cup raw cashews, well rinsed	1 teaspoon Bakon seasoning
2 tablespoons nutritional yeast flakes	½ teaspoon Vege-Sal
2 tablespoons soy sauce	½ teaspoon garlic powder
1 tablespoon canola oil	½ teaspoon ground coriander (optional)

Place all ingredients in blender and blend until smooth, approximately 3 to 4 minutes. Pour into saucepan and simmer over medium heat, stirring constantly, until mixture thickens, approximately 10 minutes. *Makes approximately 3 cups*

Creamy Oat-Mushroom Gravy

2 cups warm water	1 teaspoon Bakon seasoning
½ cup rolled oats	½ teaspoon Vege-Sal
2 tablespoons nutritional yeast flakes	½ teaspoon garlic powder
2 tablespoons soy sauce	½ teaspoon sweet basil
1 tablespoon canola oil	1 package natural mushroom-soup mix
2 teaspoons onion powder	

Place all ingredients in blender except for mushroom-soup mix. Blend until smooth, approximately 4 minutes.

Pour into saucepan and bring to a simmer over medium-low heat. Cook, stirring constantly, until mixture thickens.

Stir in mushroom-soup mix and simmer for 3 to 5 minutes more, stirring occasionally. *Makes approximately 3 cups*

Caribbean Cucumber Dressing

A cool dressing for a green salad.

1 cup Cashonnaise (page 137)

½ cup shredded cucumber

⅛ to ¼ teaspoon dried dill weed

Mix ingredients well and chill.   *Makes approximately 1½ cups*

Palm Springs Fruit Dressing

Pour this dressing over any fruit salad.

1 Cashonnaise (page 137)

1 cup unsweetened crushed pineapple, undrained

½ teaspoon ground coriander

1 ripe banana, mashed

Mix all ingredients well.   *Makes approximately 3 cups*

These recipes—quiches, a "soufflé," and a couple of delicious cookies—are presented at *the very end* of the recipes for a reason: They cannot be made without liquid egg substitute, which contains egg white. Rest assured that they are still "better for you" than recipes that are loaded with whole eggs. However, if you want to avoid *all* animal products, you may simply choose to forgo these recipes.

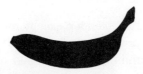

Zucchini Quiche

A traditional quiche contains eggs, cheese, and cream—a deadly trio for the blood vessels! Try this delicious alternative, which contains not a gram of cholesterol.

If you don't have time to make pie crust, buy ready-made whole-grain pie crusts from your nutrition center or health food store. Keep them in the freezer for when you want to make a "quick quiche."

1 recipe Flaky Pie Crust (page 44)	½ teaspoon salt
½ cup frozen liquid egg substitute, thawed	½ cup sliced mushrooms
1 cup Pimiento Cashew Cheese (page 135)	½ cup chopped green bell pepper
1 teaspoon ground coriander	½ cup chopped red bell pepper
½ teaspoon dried sweet basil	½ cup chopped leeks or green onions
1 teaspoon Bakon seasoning	1 cup zucchini, in thin strips
	Paprika

Preheat oven to 350°F.

Roll out half of pie crust dough and line 9-inch pie plate. (Refrigerate or freeze remaining dough to be used at another time.)

Beat egg substitute in large bowl. Stir in Pimiento Cashew Cheese, coriander, sweet basil, Bakon seasoning, and salt. Add mushrooms, bell peppers, leeks or green onions, and zucchini; mix well. Pour into pastry-lined pie plate. Sprinkle with paprika.

Bake for 45 to 50 minutes. Let set for 10 minutes before serving.

Makes 6 to 8 servings

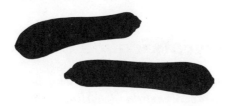

Sunflower Chili Quiche

If you don't have beans made, you may buy a 15- or 16-ounce can of vegetarian chili beans to use in this recipe instead.
  For a special treat, add 1 cup of crushed corn chips to the cheese-vegetable mixture!

½ cup frozen liquid egg
  substitute, thawed
1 cup Pimiento Cashew
  Cheese (page 135)
1 green bell pepper,
  cored, seeded, and
  chopped
1 red bell pepper, cored,
  seeded, and chopped
½ cup sliced pitted black
  olives
1 cup chopped green
  onions

1 teaspoon ground
  coriander
1 teaspoon Bakon
  seasoning
½ teaspoon salt
2 whole-wheat tortillas or
  chapati
2 cups cooked chili beans
  (see table, pages 111–
  112) or canned
½ cup shredded soy cheese
  Paprika

Preheat oven to 350°F.

Beat egg substitute in large bowl. Stir in Pimiento Cashew Cheese, bell peppers, olives, green onions, coriander, Bakon, and salt; mix well. Set aside.

Place tortillas in a 9-inch pie plate. Arrange like a sunflower, with tortilla edges curling around sides of plate.

Pour chili beans over tortillas. Pour cheese-vegetable mixture over beans. Top with the shredded soy cheese and lightly sprinkle with paprika.

Bake for 45 minutes. Let set for 10 minutes before serving.

Makes 6 to 8 servings

Veggie Scallop Quiche

Here's a quiche especially for those who would like a tasty, seafoodlike entrée. Vegetable "scallops" can be bought at a nutrition center or health food store.

1 recipe Flaky Pie Crust (page 44)

½ cup frozen liquid egg substitute, thawed

1 cup Pimiento Cashew Cheese (page 135)

1 teaspoon Bakon seasoning

1 teaspoon ground coriander

½ teaspoon dried sweet basil

½ teaspoon salt

½ cup chopped red bell pepper

½ cup sliced mushrooms

½ cup chopped leeks or green onions

1½ cups chopped vegetable scallops

Preheat oven to 350°F.

Roll out half of pie crust dough and line 9-inch pie plate. (Refrigerate or freeze remaining dough to be used at another time.)

Beat liquid egg substitute in large bowl. Stir in rest of ingredients; mix well. Pour into pastry-lined pie plate.

Bake for 40 to 45 minutes. ***Makes 6 to 8 servings***

Gourmet Cabbage Soufflé

2½ to 3 cups cooked brown rice, cooked with natural onion-soup mix added to cooking water

½ cup frozen liquid egg substitute, thawed

1 recipe Pimiento Cashew Cheese (page 135)

1 teaspoon ground coriander

1 teaspoon Bakon seasoning

1 teaspoon dried sweet basil

½ teaspoon salt

2 cups shredded Chinese or celery cabbage

1 cup chopped green onions

1 cup chopped green bell pepper

½ cup whole-grain cracker crumbs, onion-flavored if possible

Preheat oven to 350°F.

Press cooked brown rice firmly over bottom of a 13 x 9-inch baking dish.

Beat liquid egg substitute in large bowl. Stir in Pimiento Cashew Cheese, coriander, Bakon, sweet basil, and salt; add cabbage, green onions, and bell pepper and mix well. Pour mixture over rice. Top with cracker crumbs.

Bake for 45 minutes. Let set a few minutes before serving.

Makes 10 servings

Mandarin Rangers

Cookies are a special challenge for the cook who wants to use wholesome ingredients—specifically, their texture is a challenge. How do you get a crisp or crunchy cookie when the shortening is oil, the flour is whole wheat, and the sweetening is honey or banana?

You can meet the challenge by using crunchy, whole-grain flaked cereal as a major ingredient. (Be sure you buy a whole-grain brand. There are several good brands carried by health food stores; some grocery stores stock them, too, but be sure to choose a brand with little or no sugar.) The texture is very satisfying, that special combination of chewy and crisp that most people like in cookies—and the flavor is delightful.

One caution: Just as certain brands of cereal can get soggy in milk, they make your cookies go soft after a day or so. To be sure they stay crisp, store them in the refrigerator and take them out as needed. If you have children in the house, there's a good chance there won't be any left after the first day!

2 cups whole-grain flaked cereal
1 cup whole-wheat flour
1 cup rolled oats
½ cup chopped pecans
½ cup finely shredded unsweetened coconut
½ cup carob chips (sweetened with dates or barley malt)
½ cup canola oil
½ cup honey

¼ cup frozen liquid egg substitute, thawed
2 tablespoons frozen orange juice concentrate, thawed
1 teaspoon ground coriander
½ teaspoon orange extract
½ teaspoon salt
½ teaspoon almond extract
½ teaspoon grated orange peel

Preheat oven to 375°F.

In large bowl mix together cereal, flour, oats, pecans, coconut, and carob chips.

Place remaining ingredients in small bowl or in blender and blend well. Pour this liquid mixture over dry ingredients and mix with spoon or hands until all is evenly moistened. Drop by large spoonfuls onto cookie sheets lined with waxed paper.

Bake for 12 to 15 minutes or until brown on bottom.

Makes approximately 2 dozen cookies

Nutty Buddies

These cookies are similar in some way to those in the preceding recipe, though some children may prefer them because they have a "plainer" flavor—no orange or almond. Their dominant flavor is that of toasted nuts—scrumptious!

2 cups whole-grain flaked cereal
1 cup whole-wheat flour
1 cup rolled oats
½ cup chopped pecans
½ cup finely shredded unsweetened coconut
1 cup raisins
¼ cup raw sunflower seeds

½ cup canola oil
½ cup honey
¼ cup frozen liquid egg substitute, thawed
1 teaspoon ground coriander
2 teaspoons vanilla extract
½ teaspoon salt

Preheat oven to 375°F.

In large bowl mix together cereal, flour, oats, pecans, coconut, raisins, and sunflower seeds.

Place remaining ingredients in small bowl or in blender and beat or blend thoroughly. Pour this liquid mixture over dry ingredients and mix with spoon or hands until all is evenly moistened. Drop by large spoonfuls onto cookie sheets lined with waxed paper.

Bake for 12 to 15 minutes or until brown on bottom.

Makes approximately 2 dozen cookies

WORKING THE PROGRAM

A *diet high in fat almost invariably results in a body high in fat.* Much human suffering and disease has been linked to the fat in our diets.

Most of the time we may be convinced of this fact. But when we are faced with a savory meal loaded with cheese or with a buttery dessert, it's hard to make the connection between food and disease. How can something so delicious be deadly?

But more and more people are making the connection and are trying to give up harmful fats. Along the way they have found that new ways of eating aren't all that bad. There are delicious whole-grain breads to discover, savory and filling beans and pasta, and a tremendous and colorful variety of produce.

But let's face it. One thing about those troubling fats: They *taste* good! A minimal-fat diet *can* be bleak unless careful planning is given to flavor.

As you begin to explore cooking Adventist-style, you'll notice that one way Adventists build flavor into their recipes is by using nuts, seeds, even avocados and coconut.

But wait, you may think—aren't those foods high in fat? The first thing to remember is that the fats these foods contain are nature's fats, and come complete with vitamins, minerals, fiber, and protein. It is true that avocados and coconut contain large amounts of palmitic and lauric acid, which raise blood cholesterol levels. However, animal studies have shown that if there is no cholesterol in the diet, animals can take in large quantities of coconut without developing atherosclerosis. We may conclude that total vegetarians will have no problem in using coconut or avocados. Nuts, although high in fat, are not high in the types of fatty acids that elevate blood cholesterol. An interesting bit of recent information comes from a large study of Seventh-Day Adventists: those who ate nuts daily had a heart attack rate that was *half* that of those who ate nuts rarely!

The "killer" fats, those that are truly unhealthful and should be eliminated as far as possible, include butter, animal fats, hydrogenated oils. It is important to note that at present Seventh-Day Adventists are eating as much fat as people in the general population

(37 percent), and yet they have less than half the deaths from heart attacks and even from cancers that are unrelated to alcohol and tobacco. The type of fat consumed is at least as important as the amount of fat consumed. More fat would not necessarily harm you if it was all from plant sources.

The best news for dieters who miss creamy sauces and mayonnaise is the cashew. Do cashews belong in a weight-loss program? Salted cashews, roasted in oil, certainly do not, but raw cashews are a wonderful way to add flavor and texture to a healthy diet. Because they are soft, when placed in a blender with other ingredients and seasonings, they make sauces with a wonderful creamy texture. Try Pimiento Cashew Cheese (page 135) and Cashonnaise (page 137) and you will not feel deprived.

Of course, one must exercise moderation even with these naturally good fats. The largest part of the diet should still be fresh fruits and vegetables, grains, and legumes. Nuts, seeds, avocados, and coconut are important for flavor and nutrition, but should not be eaten in large quantities—just enough for flavor and satisfaction!

You will notice that some of the recipes in this book contain a little oil—olive oil or canola oil, both of which are of benefit to those watching their cholesterol levels. Olive oil is unique in that it helps keep the arteries elastic by its action on the artery walls; canola oil helps keep the blood from clotting, and in this way reduces heart attack risk. Corn, safflower, and sunflower oils are other good oils; they help to lower blood cholesterol. But we recommend keeping these visible fats to a minimum, and those who want to speed up their weight loss and those who are recovering from illness will want to cut back on them as far as possible. See Chapter 2 for other ideas on flavoring vegetables the low-fat way.

As you have seen, vegetarians who follow an Adventist life-style have an even more impressive record of health and longevity than nonvegetarian Adventists. But please don't despair if you are not ready to give up all meat and dairy products. Remember that *every step you take* toward health will do you good. An "all-or-nothing" mentality is the way to defeat. Perhaps you'll decide to cut out cheese but still drink skim milk; perhaps you have eliminated beef and pork from your diet, but still eat chicken and fish. Chicken and fish are better than the red meats because they have less saturated fat. However, chicken contains as much cholesterol as beef. Even 3½ ounces of fish contains 40 to 60 milligrams of cholesterol and thus cannot be considered a low-cholesterol food. The oxidation products of fish fats may be cancer-producing. Elimination of red meats is the first step to better health and may cut your heart attack risk in half, but elimination of fish and poultry may reduce it by half again.

Start by making the changes that you feel comfortable with. Once you notice how good you've begun to feel, you'll want to make even more changes.

· S U M M A R Y ·

1. Coronary heart disease is the most common cause of death in the United States.

2. The most powerful and most financially sound way to treat heart disease is through *prevention*. This calls for a drastic reduction of cholesterol and saturated fat in the diet. Cholesterol is found only in animal products; harmful dietary fats are saturated *animal* fats.

3. A number of studies indicate that the progression of atherosclerosis can be reversed.

4. A vegetarian diet can substantially lower the serum cholesterol level.

5. A sudden change to a vegetarian diet is usually not the best way. It's better to begin slowly, eating more fruits, vegetables, grains, and legumes, and gradually deemphasizing the role of meat in the diet.

• This Week's Guide to Success •

Make a conscious effort to reduce dietary fat.

Begin substituting natural plant-fat alternative recipes for empty-calorie, high-fat foods—e.g., nut or fruit butters for butter or margarine, Cashonnaise (page 137) for mayonnaise, Pimiento Cashew Cheese (page 135) for cheese.

If you eat meat at almost every meal, begin to experiment with meatless meals a few times a week.

Substitute vegetarian entrées for meat dishes, using the recipes in this book or creating your own.

Eat slowly and chew your food thoroughly.

This will increase your enjoyment of the meal as well as provide nutritional benefits by aiding digestion. Remember, when you begin to eat more fiber and less fat, you will be eating foods that require more chewing. Slow down!

Observe how satisfied you're beginning to feel.

Fiber-rich whole foods have more bulk, which makes them more satisfying than animal products or refined foods, because they fill your stomach even though they are low in calories.

5

· *Principle No. 5* ·

The Fast

*. . . most persons who give the plan a trial, will
find that two meals a day are better than three.*
—*Ellen G. White*

I t may seem a little strange, but there *are* people who fast regularly and with enthusiasm. There are also a lot of us who have
tried fasting and have ended up with shaky knees, an unpleasant
disposition, and a tendency to gorge once the fast is broken!

The Seventh-Day Adventist way of fasting insists on no extremes.
It makes allowances for the fact that what may be safe and beneficial
for one person may be too severe for another. It allows eating enough
nourishing food at nonfasting times so that when you do fast, you
don't feel weak and desperate. Seventh-Day Adventists see fasting
as a time of rest and recovery for the body—and also as a powerful
instrument for weight loss and weight control.

This is the principle that makes this program different from other
weight-loss plans you have seen. It allows you the pleasure of eating
satisfying meals, and also ensures that a large part of your day will
be spent burning calories.

You can get used to the idea of fasting by recognizing that you
already fast for a number of hours—at night, while you sleep. The
plan is to extend your fasting time into the waking hours of the day.

The Seventh-Day Adventist plan prescribes two main meals per
day (breakfast and lunch), and an optional light supper. In between,
you take in nothing but water. No snacks!

Cutting out snacks, of course, is not a revolutionary idea. It is
common to many diets of the "sensible" type. Unfortunately, many of
these "sensible" diets allow a breakfast of, say, dry toast, coffee, and
half a grapefruit. For lunch you may—if you're lucky—be allowed
"three ounces of tuna, a teaspoon of mayonnaise, a slice of diet bread,
and an apple."

After a spartan regime such as this, it is no wonder the theory that it is better to eat many meals during the day was greeted with such relief! The idea that snacking is "good for you," that you can eat all day long "and *still* lose weight," holds an irresistible appeal for people who have been schooled on deprivation. People like to eat!

But there are several big problems with eating many meals throughout the day. One is that they must necessarily be *very small* meals. You are always living on the edge of hunger. Another problem is that you may become preoccupied with thoughts of food. This is especially likely to happen if none of the meals allows you to eat to satisfaction. Many of us have been known to eat for solace, entertainment, and other reasons that have little to do with hunger. Feeling a burden to eat six to eight times a day may actually feed the problem known as food addiction. It cannot be denied that there is an emotional component to compulsive eating—but sometimes the problem simply "disappears" when a person learns to eat a substantial, nutritious breakfast and a substantial, nutritious lunch.

Many busy people are convinced they don't have time to sit down to a real meal. They might be pleasantly surprised to find that if they eat two good meals, the rest of the day is theirs, to do their work, to exercise, to talk, to play. If your work requires lots of concentration, it is better not to have to think too much about food. If you need to take occasional breaks, it is far better to take a walk or a telephone break than to take a snack break.

If you are used to depending on snacks to get you through the day, you may find yourself getting very hungry when you cut them out. The answer is not to give in to snacking, but to make sure you are eating enough for breakfast and lunch. An especially troublesome time may be late afternoon, when many people experience a noticeable drop in "blood sugar"—and an increase in irritability that unfortunately may also be quite noticeable! Dealing with these "low times" with coffee and sugary snacks will in the long run worsen the problem. But so strong is the desire to feel good (and a perfectly reasonable desire it is!) that we may gratefully welcome the temporary lift that comes from sugar and caffeine.

Your ultimate goal, of course, is to have the greatest energy, health, and well-being possible, and "quick fixes" of snacks, especially unhealthful snacks, will sabotage this goal. Please try eating a good breakfast and a good lunch (perhaps later in the day than you are used to, at one or two o'clock), and see if you can go the entire afternoon without a snack.

Seventh-Day Adventists believe that eating two meals a day, with an optional light third meal, is better for the digestive system and body processes. The stomach needs periods of rest, for digestion is real work. Going to bed with undigested food in the stomach may turn the process of digestion into a kind of putrefaction and often results in bad breath and bad health. Seventh-Day Adventists also believe that eating the bulk of one's calories in the evening can lead to obesity.

There are studies that indicate that eating just two meals a day can indeed make losing weight easier. Studies published in the 1960s found that obese people who are unable to stick to traditional low-calorie diets are more successful when put on diets of the same number of calories divided between two meals rather than three. The researchers suggested that the two-meal-a-day plan was easier to adhere to both because there was less exposure to food and because the larger meals did not leave the patients hungry: "It is remarkable that obese patients who have failed to lose weight when taking food several times a day can lose weight when their meals are reduced to two a day though the total *prescribed calories* remain the same."

We certainly know that eating fewer meals is better for our teeth! Snacking between meals is the cause of much tooth decay.

The two meals should be substantial. On this plan you do not count calories—but if you *were* to calculate the number of calories needed to maintain your ideal weight, you would divide them between these two meals.

This is not a diet plan that makes you feel as if you are starving. What is important is *what* you eat (low-fat, whole-grain, fresh, delicious foods) and *when* you eat.

Many people will find that by eating two meals in the first half of the day, they are not even hungry for dinner, or they feel a mild kind of hunger that is easily tolerable. If you are not too uncomfortable, you may go without dinner entirely. Thus you have extended your fast from lunch to breakfast of the following day. Sometimes you may feel a hunger that is fairly sharp, but if you wait a little, or drink a glass or two of water, hunger pangs may fade away.

However—if you feel nauseated, extremely grouchy, faint, or very weak, by all means have a light supper of fruit and whole grains. This does not mean that you are "off the plan." It still allows for satisfactory weight loss and good health.

This light supper is not a bedtime snack, nor is it a midnight snack. It should be eaten several hours before bedtime. Some people who have been on very austere weight-loss programs cannot imagine going to bed without eating at least a few crackers to prevent hunger pangs from keeping them awake. This is not necessary on this program! In fact, it would slow down your weight loss considerably. It is necessary for health and weight loss to go to bed with an empty stomach—and what makes that possible are the two meals you will have eaten earlier in the day.

Here is a complete Menu Planner to help with your daily food choices. So that you can get a good idea of what the average day will be like, we have repeated the basics of the breakfast plan that was more fully explained in Chapter 1.

Menu Planner

Water: One or two 8-ounce glasses

BREAKFAST

1 slice whole-grain bread

1 teaspoon nut butter

½ to 1 cup whole-grain cereal or other protein food

1 citrus fruit

1 other fruit

1 glass (8 ounces) milk

Water: Two 8-ounce glasses

LUNCH

1 entrée

1 green leafy vegetable

1 other vegetable

1 raw vegetable salad

1 slice whole-grain bread

1 glass (8 ounces) milk

Water: Two 8-ounce glasses

S U P P E R *(if eaten)*

1 fruit

1 slice whole-grain bread or
3 to 4 whole-grain crackers

Water: Two 8-ounce glasses

For lunch:

One entrée: The entrée should be high in protein and low in fat. It may be based on a legume (served alone or with rice or whole-grain pasta), a vegetable protein product such as tofu, or a high-protein grain. If you are still eating animal protein, please choose the leaner kinds—fish or chicken as opposed to beef or pork.

One green leafy vegetable: Choose from kale, broccoli, collards, mustard greens, spinach, beet greens, Swiss chard, etc.

One other vegetable: Choose from potato, carrots, eggplant, squash, asparagus, sweet potato, cauliflower, beets, cabbage, green beans, sweet peas, etc.

One raw vegetable salad: Vary the recipes for your salads. Try serving with lemon juice and herbs or small amounts of healthful salad dressing—or eat a raw vegetable instead.

One slice whole-grain bread: A plain toasted slice of good whole-grain bread goes well with a savory entrée. Or dice the toasted bread and serve as croutons on your salad.

One glass (8 ounces) milk: Skim milk, soy milk, nut milk, cultured buttermilk, or lowfat yogurt.

For supper:

It is desirable to choose a different fruit from what you had for breakfast. If you are very hungry, eat more than one fruit!

It is recommended that you stick fairly closely to the Menu Planner, at least at first, so you can begin to experience how *much* food is the appropriate amount. Later, when you have a pretty good idea of what the plan is all about, you don't have to be so rigid—only reasonable. (For example, don't give up your spinach in order to have an extra helping of dessert!)

Most people who follow this eating plan closely will feel better, have more energy, and happily lose weight. There are some who should exercise a little care, however, when thinking about eliminating the third meal. Those who have been diagnosed as hypoglycemic or diabetic and others with chronic conditions should consult their doctors, who will more than likely advise that the third meal be retained in some form.

Ellen White herself found great benefits in eating two meals a day, and saw the plan benefit many others, but she did not bind family and guests with rigid rules. She wrote, "Our table is set twice a day, but if there are those who desire something to eat in the evening, there is no rule that forbids them from getting it. No one complains or goes from our table dissatisfied." This is especially applicable to children, whose metabolic needs may be different from those of adults. It is a good idea to keep granola, bread, fruit, and leftovers in the kitchen for children who are hungry after school or in the evening.

But there is no rule that says that parents must wait on children at every meal! Many parents who willingly provide two nourishing meals in the first part of the day would like freedom from kitchen chores in the afternoon and evening. These are the times when children may serve themselves.

There is another group, a *small* group, of people who should also modify the eating plan: These are the people who spend much of their day doing hard physical work. They will still benefit from eating low-fat, fresh, whole food—they will just eat more of it! An early evening meal may be a necessity for someone who has burned thousands of calories during the day.

Along with any fast, or any weight-loss plan, you must drink water. *Lots* of water.

One of the body's remarkable functions is the cleansing and regulating function of the kidneys. The kidneys require a generous amount of water, as they produce an average of 200 *liters* of filtrate each day. (They don't require an *intake* of 200 liters of water, fortunately—six to eight glasses daily will do the job!) They are designed so that if not enough water is supplied, they will pull water from the large intestine and other tissues. A person will generally survive if the kidneys are called upon to do this, but anyone interested enough to read this book probably has goals that go beyond simple survival; goals like feeling good, looking good, and achieving optimum health! We are more likely to reach these goals if we don't ask the kidneys to work overtime and if we provide them with the water needed to efficiently cleanse the body of wastes.

We recommend that you drink six to eight glasses of fresh, pure water each day.

Many people who significantly increase the amount of water they drink report improvements in their skin, in its clarity, texture, and softness. Drinking lots of water also helps to eliminate snacking. Sometimes when we think we need food what we really need is a glass or two of fresh water, and the craving for food will subside. Because we feel better when we are well hydrated, we may not be as tempted to "cheat" with sugary foods. Please note that a soft drink is no substitute for a glass of fresh water. Soft drinks between meals increase the flow of gastric juice 3½ to 5 times as much as does water. The stomach should not be pushed to produce gastric juice all day long! The ideal beverage is water—and most of us don't get nearly as much of it as we should.

Finally we come to the "secret weapon": a day-long, total fast. This is especially for people who have a great deal of weight to lose or who are eager to lose weight in a hurry.

There are many books written on fasting techniques and the benefits of fasting, and it is beyond the scope of this book to go deeply into the subject. Suffice it to say that Seventh-Day Adventists believe fasting has incalculable benefits: in cleansing the body, in allowing the digestive system to rest, in helping to cure illness, and in strengthening the character.

The day-long, total fast is presented in this book as an aid to reducing. It is perfectly safe for the healthy person who is not hypoglycemic or diabetic to abstain from food one day a week. As long as you stick to the Menu Planner the other six days, the speed with which you will lose weight will be gratifying.

The most extreme way of experiencing the day-long fast is to drink only water. Be sure to drink *plenty* of water!

If this is too severe for you, you may drink natural juices (such as carrot, apple, grape) and eat fresh fruit throughout the day, or even eat *very lightly* of other types of wholesome foods. Just be sure that you don't skimp on water!

If you feel you are not ready for a total fast, remember that you are already experiencing some of the benefits of fasting if you have eliminated snacking between meals and/or have eliminated the evening meal. Ellen White herself wrote that the true fast is "abstinence from every stimulating kind of food, and the proper use of wholesome, simple food . . ." This suggests an understanding of fasting not as a denial of all substances, but as a refusal to take any *harmful* substances into the body.

• WORKING THE • PROGRAM

If you are having difficulties getting in your full six to eight glasses of water every day, there are some things you can do to make it easier. If you suspect your tap water contains impurities, you may want to buy bottled water in jugs, the kind with a spout near the bottom for easy dispensing, and keep one on your countertop at all times. (Many people don't need a lab test to discover how unsuitable their tap water is; their eyes, nose, and taste buds tell them they should use purified water for cooking as well as for drinking.) We have discovered that we can save about two-thirds on the cost of water if we fill our own jugs when we purchase filtered water.

Some people don't like to have to think about sipping water all day long and would rather drink several glasses at once. It's easier to do this if the water is not too cold, perhaps kept in a jug on the countertop in the kitchen, or in a bottle at work. Simply make sure that you drink water four times a day:

1 to 2 glasses before breakfast

2 glasses in the morning

2 glasses in the afternoon

2 glasses in the evening

If you prefer cold water, by all means drink it cold. However, Seventh-Day Adventists often recommend room-temperature water because they believe it is more readily utilized in the body—especially good after heavy exercise or on hot days.

You may come up with your own ideas to make sure you get your six to eight glasses. You may carry to work a container that holds the entire amount of water you should drink for the day—just make sure you have drunk it by the end of the day! Carry a cup of water with you whenever you can, into classes if you are a student, into business meetings, in your car in a holder that hooks onto the side window. The lidded containers with spouts that bicyclists carry with them are most convenient for some people.

One Seventh-Day Adventist health educator devoted part of a nutrition class to the importance of drinking lots of water. A woman raised her hand and objected: "But if I drink that much water, I'll have to go to the bathroom more!"

The teacher gave her a frank and friendly stare and said: "Then go to the bathroom more."

A flippant reply, perhaps—but the point is that if it requires more frequent urination to keep the kidneys in good working order, to keep the skin in good condition, and to help maintain ideal weight, then it is worth it. Many people pay for the "convenience" of infrequent trips to the bathroom with frequent bladder infections—and there is nothing convenient about a bladder infection!

This "fasting" principle is a favorite because it is the one that speeds weight loss. It is indeed thrilling to know that if you put on a few extra pounds there's no need to panic or to worry about losing control. Skipping the evening meal is the *surefire* way to maintain weight loss. The other six principles are significant, of course, but we emphasize this one because in many ways it is the key to losing weight with ease. It is hard to express the satisfaction that a life-long dieter feels at being able to sit down to a big breakfast, and again to a substantial lunch, without guilt. With the evening comes another kind of satisfaction, at feeling light but not frantic, at being aware of a flattening stomach, at knowing there will be no penalty to pay for a delicious breakfast and lunch.

At first, however, you may find this the most difficult principle to follow. You may believe that there is no way you can eliminate your evening meal. This, indeed, was Jan's most difficult challenge. Late afternoon was her "low" time of the day, and she was convinced the only way she could battle her fatigue was with food.

Chris persuaded her to try eating only a plateful of fruit in the evening, as fruit is easily digested, with little expenditure of energy. After a day or so of this she was stunned to realize that she was *less* tired than usual. When she woke up in the morning she was clear-headed and did not feel her usual desperation for an immediate breakfast. The very thing she thought was saving her from faintness and tiredness (eating food at night) was actually contributing to the problem!

In Ellen G. White's writings is a description of the very process Jan went through when she was trying to eliminate the evening meal:

Those who are changing from three meals a day, to two, will at first be troubled more or less with faintness, especially about the time they have been in the habit of eating their third meal. But if they persevere for a short time, this faintness will disappear.

. . . The work of digestion should not be carried on through any period of the sleeping hours. After the stomach, which has been overtaxed, has performed its task, it becomes exhausted, which causes faintness. Here many are deceived, and think that it is the want of food which produces such feelings, and without giving the stomach time to rest, they take more food, which for the time removes the faintness. And the more the appetite is indulged, the more will be its clamors for gratification. This faintness is generally the result of meat eating, and eating frequently, and too much. The stomach becomes weary by being kept constantly at work, disposing of food not the most healthful. Having no time for rest, the digestive organs become enfeebled, hence the sense of "goneness," and desire for frequent eating. The remedy such require, is to eat less frequently and less liberally, and be satisfied with plain, simple food, eating twice, or, at most, three times a day. . . .

Jan has since found by experimentation that when she eats at night she has more trouble controlling her weight; when she returns to a fruit-only evening snack, she slims down very quickly.

Often we attribute compulsive eating to purely emotional factors, but compulsive behavior is sometimes the body's desperate attempt to find nutrients it needs. With the improvement in nutrition that will result from the SDA program, you will find you have less of a desire to overeat.

Of course there are other reasons for eating disorders, such as depression, anxiety, and other emotional or mental causes, which may be best dealt with through professional therapy. However, we are convinced that these cases are fewer in number than most people think and that changes in life-style will take care of many eating problems. In Chapter 7 you will find ideas for alleviating the milder forms of stress and anxiety that often undermine our attempts to take care of our bodies and to enjoy them in full.

And now to discuss the most troublesome aspect of changing to a healthy new way of life—that is, social pressure. All other obstacles seem to pale by comparison—especially if you are accustomed to eating out in the evening, entertaining business associates, or cooking for friends at home. We don't want to minimize the problem, but we do want to suggest some ways of making it less difficult.

Most important is convincing yourself that you will feel better and lose weight more easily by having a light evening meal or none at all. Once you have experienced the plan for a week or two or a month you will genuinely feel better, and you will be motivated to find a way to fit it into your life forever.

Please remember that many people use special diets as an excuse to eat differently from those around them. For the first few weeks on the plan you may wish to excuse yourself on such grounds; later, you might want to think of another tactic. Skipping dinner as a weight-loss measure is not so weird as you may think and is getting more common, even among people who have never heard of a Seventh-Day Adventist plan for health. At some evening functions you can get away with eating fruit and no one will even notice. Most people will understand if you ask for a simple salad at dinner. (If you must eat in the evening, fruit is better than salad, but salad is much better than steak!)

One woman was convinced that this plan could never work, because the evening meal was the only time she and her husband had to spend some time together. Her husband pointed out that they would have *more* time together if she weren't in the kitchen cooking dinner, and suggested they eat a simple plate of fruit in the evening.

Once the desired amount of weight has been lost, some people will want to make an occasional exception to the plan (though the longer you follow the plan, the better you will feel, and the less you will *want* to make exceptions). It usually is possible to choose something acceptable from food that is offered to you. Be sure to praise the fruit, vegetables, and other good food that you select—a little charm may inspire your host or hostess to prepare the foods you like in the future!

Of course the easiest way to make these changes is to socialize with people who are interested in making the same changes—if your life-style allows it, get together for lunch or breakfast, or serve special fruit drinks or fruit desserts for evening get-togethers. If you are entertaining friends who are used to eating more in the evening, you will, of course, offer them more than you yourself may eat.

The good news is that the world is making it easier for a health-conscious person to follow healthful eating practices. The number of health-conscious people is rising; people are becoming more tolerant of "new" ways of eating; and, more specifically, more people are placing a greater emphasis on breakfast and eating lightly in the evening.

• S U M M A R Y •

1. A time of fasting is a time of rest and recovery for the body and is also a powerful instrument for weight control.

2. The Seventh-Day Adventist plan for health and weight loss prescribes breakfast, lunch, and an optional light supper, with nothing taken between meals except water.

3. Trying to eat many small meals throughout the day may exaggerate problems with compulsive eating, will overtax the digestive system, and in many cases will make losing weight more difficult.

4. Calories ingested in the evening will result in inefficient digestion, may elevate serum cholesterol and triglycerides, and may lead to obesity.

5. Studies show that eating only two meals a day (skipping dinner, not breakfast) can make losing weight easier.

6. The optional light supper of fruit and whole grains should be eaten at least three to five hours before bedtime.

7. Drinking six to eight glasses of fresh, pure water each day is essential in maintaining health and losing weight.

8. A day-long, total fast is an option for those who want to lose weight quickly.

• This Week's Guide to Success •

Cut out snacks.
  Eat only at mealtimes, at the kitchen or dining room table.

Drink six to eight glasses of water daily.
  Follow the simple fluid schedule. When you're tempted to snack, drink a glass or two of water.

Deemphasize the evening meal.
  If you can't cut out the evening meal entirely, make sure it is a light one, eaten at least three to five hours before bedtime. One night this week, try going without this meal; if you get hungry, eat some fruit.

Consider the day-long fast.
  Those without hypoglycemia or diabetes or other medical conditions that would preclude it might try fasting one full day this week. Be sure to drink plenty of fluids as described in this chapter.

6

· *Principle No. 6* ·

Exercise

*Inactivity is a fruitful cause of disease. Exercise
quickens and equalizes the circulation of the
blood, but in idleness the blood does not
circulate freely, and the changes in it, so
necessary to life and health, do not take place.*
—Ellen G. White

According to a 1989 poll conducted by American Sports Data,
Inc., 42 million Americans over the age of six participate in a
sporting event or other physical workout at least one hundred days
out of the year. This is encouraging—but it still leaves a sizable
number of people who are missing out on one of the real joys of life!

The most difficult problem in following an exercise program tends
to be that of motivation. For many people the best solution to the
problem is to combine exercise with sociability. If you know someone
is counting on you to go for a run or a jog, that's an incentive for you
to keep the running date. For many people who have begun a walking
program, the fun is magnified by sharing it with a friend, or with a
whole group of friends. (It is an advantage to your weight-loss program if you can learn to talk and walk briskly at the same time!)
Once your level of fitness is up, you may want to learn a sport, or to
take classes in swimming or aerobics. Sometimes when you're having
fun, exertion seems almost effortless.

Choose your companions carefully. If you are a beginner, working
out with an advanced athlete or with one who is very competitive can
demoralize you. It is good if those who run or walk or play tennis
together are either well matched in physical condition and skill, or
are very patient with one another.

We're not suggesting that you hide away to avoid competition. It is

165

sad how many people will not learn a sport or walk or lift weights because someone might "see" them! We are only suggesting that you avoid adding unnecessary pressure, and make working out as much fun as possible.

It might help to motivate you if you know some of the advantages of a regular exercise program.

First, it is extremely difficult to lose weight or to maintain one's "dream weight" without exercising. Dieting without exercise usually means a food program that is so austere that much of the fun is taken out of life. Such a spartan diet puts you in danger of not getting all the nutrients that are necessary for health and a feeling of well-being. (A feeling of well-being is something else that helps make life fun!) A regular exercise program makes very low calorie diets unnecessary for most people.

As exercise helps to normalize your weight, it will also help keep at bay certain deadly diseases: diabetes, osteoporosis, cancer, and diseases of the heart and blood vessels. It helps prevent some diabetes because it controls weight and improves the ability of receptor cells to utilize insulin; it clearly plays an important role in preventing osteoporosis; and its role in reducing the risk of cancer comes from its weight-control function. Exercise helps control cholesterol levels in two ways. One is through its simple weight-controlling function. The other has to do with its effect on the ratio of high-density lipoproteins (HDLs) to low-density lipoproteins (LDLs) in the blood. HDLs are the "good" type of cholesterol that helps prevent the buildup of fatty deposits by removing the bad kind of cholesterol from the bloodstream. LDLs, in contrast, form dangerous deposits on the walls of blood vessels and can cause clogged arteries and atherosclerosis. All the fitness-minded person really needs to know about these lipoproteins is that the higher the ratio of HDLs to LDLs in the blood, the lower the risk of heart disease—and regular exercise generally *raises* the level of HDLs. It must be noted that one must walk three miles a day, five days a week, before one can expect changes in the level of HDLs. A little exercise now and then won't do it.

Exercise is also wonderful for relieving stress and "clearing the mental circuits." A brisk walk or swim or game of tennis can noticeably brighten your spirits.

A recent study shows that even a little exercise can measurably increase longevity. In fact, new research shows that the greatest health improvements come from exercising enough to get out of the "sedentary" category. And exercise will help to alleviate some of the disastrous results that may come from those times you do *not* adhere to the rest of the health principles.

For a time some exercise specialists thought that if one exercised enough it would not be necessary to watch one's diet. Dr. Kenneth Cooper of aerobics fame now states this is wrong. Even with a good exercise program, hardening of the arteries will continue to progress if you do not eat right. Diet and exercise are equally important.

Sometimes in an Adventist health class someone will raise his or her hand and say: "My grandfather ate three heavy meals a day, lots of butter and white flour and pork, and he lived to be a hundred and three!"

This person's grandfather also lived on a farm and did hard physical labor from sunup to sundown. Physical exercise will make up for some deficiencies in diet, but it is important to remember that it is very rare nowadays to be able to exercise as hard as our ancestors did. (It is also good to realize that Grandfather also got lots of fresh air and probably lots of fresh vegetables—and that if he had left out the white flour and pork, maybe he would have lived to be a hundred and six!)

An exercise program can make a significant contribution to a good self-image. Knowing that you are at your physical best increases your self-confidence. It helps you acquire poise and grace, which improve the appearance and are also helpful in social situations.

Some call exercise the fountain of youth. We know one woman in her sixties who, from a distance, looks like a girl. Her back is straight, her stomach flat, her motions fluid, body slim. The lines on her face are largely from laughter. Though she also pays attention to the rest of the principles that promote health, it is her enthusiasm for exercise that has resulted in her youthful appearance.

And the men who maintain that "aura of youth," avoiding the softening that often comes with age, are those who have continued to exercise!

Good muscle tone is essential for good posture, and both can help with avoiding the back pain that tends to plague many who lead sedentary lives.

One reason sustained exercise results in greater energy is that it provides the muscle tissues with more oxygen. It also increases the number and size of the mitochondria, which are what produce the energy in the cells. It has also been suggested that it slows down the aging process and reduces the likelihood of getting cancer. A person who exercises regularly will sleep better and will get more work done with less fatigue.

Having proclaimed the virtues of exercise in general, let us take a look at the Seventh-Day Adventist specialty: walking.

Walking is a favorite of Adventists, who like to exercise in the open air, back straight, breathing deeply. If your day is stressful and chaotic, a long walk will provide serenity and relief. If you feel sluggish after a long day at your desk, a brisk walk will provide stimulation. Adventists regard walking in the fresh air as a fine recreational activity to do with family and friends, and also consider a moderate walk after a meal to aid in the digestive process.

Walking may be the very best activity for most people. It is easier on the joints than running, and it is more difficult to injure oneself while walking than while doing most other sports. It is inexpensive, requiring only a good pair of walking shoes; and many people need only step out the front door to take a walk. A decade ago it was more common to see joggers and runners taking the air; these days a larger percentage of health-minded people seem to be walking. All persons aged thirty-five and older should be checked by a physician before any vigorous exercise is attempted. Your doctor may even suggest that an electrocardiogram stress test be performed first. However, walking is a safe exercise and can be graduated. This is the exercise that is best recommended for most people.

For good health and weight loss the walking pace should be *brisk*. To help you work up to a good fat-burning pace we have included a walking chart at the end of this chapter.

A word of caution: It is possible to be engaged in an excellent walking program, to be slim, and to have a healthy heart and the bloom that comes from exercise—and still experience some stiffness. This is likely to occur if you don't do any stretching of your body. Walking is wonderful, and some people seem to thrive on walking alone. But if you want a taut stomach, a feeling of strength and straightness in your spine, and a more shapely body, some good stretches are in order—along with some modified sit-ups.

There are good reasons to stretch: Stretching induces relaxation, helps coordination by allowing free movement, and helps prevent injuries. A strong prestretched muscle resists stress better than a strong *un*stretched muscle. Stretching promotes circulation—and it *feels good*.

Stretching does not mean that you force your body into uncomfortable or painful positions. Stretching motions should be slow, controlled, and carried to the point where the stretch is felt—but they should *not* cause pain. If you are not limber, a small stretch will do as much for your body as a larger stretch will do for someone who is more limber. Also, be sure to keep your knees slightly bent at all times in order to avoid injuring your back. The importance of protecting your back should not be underestimated—it is suspected that eight out of ten people have back problems at some time.

From a fitness instructor, an athletic friend, or an exercise book you can learn some wonderful, thorough stretches. Here we give you a "bare-minimum" routine that will help prevent injuries if you do it before and after exercise and will also give your muscles a little extra tone.

1. Tilt ear toward shoulder while pressing both shoulders down. Relax neck, lowering chin to chest. Repeat on other side. Do both sides slowly, 5 times.

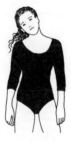

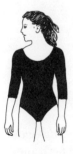

2. Gently turn head so that chin is over one shoulder. Shoulders should remain still. Slowly turn head from side to side 5 times.

3. Standing, reach to front with straight arms and clasp hands in front of shoulders. Tuck chin to chest and gently press arms away from body, rounding shoulders and back. Repeat 5 times.

4. Standing, place one hand on waist for support, then reach straight up with other arm. Repeat this reaching motion 10 times on each side (do more repetitions as desired, reaching higher and higher for a trimmer waist).

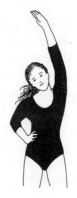

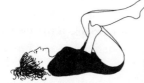

5. Lie on back on floor, knees bent and feet flat. Relax neck and shoulders. Place both hands under thighs and pull knees toward chest. Return knees to floor. Repeat slowly 10 times.

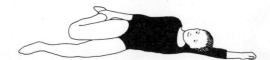

6. Roll to one side, head resting on outstretched arm on floor, both knees bent forward. Grasp ankle of upper leg with hand and pull gently backward, *without arching back*. Repeat 5 times, then roll to other side and do 5 repetitions on other leg.

7. Lie on back, head and shoulders relaxed, knees bent and feet flat on floor. Place hands under right thigh and gently pull right knee toward chest. Slowly extend right leg, flexing foot, until you feel a mild stretch. Return foot to floor and repeat with left leg. Alternate 5 times.

8. Stand with one leg approximately 18 inches in front of the other, toes pointed forward. Keep back heel on floor and slowly lean forward, resting hands on thigh of front leg, until you feel a mild tension in calf muscle of rear leg. Hold for a count of 10 and release. Repeat 5 times on each side.

Strong abdominal muscles will help prevent back pain and will also help with any physical activity. For the much neglected but very important abdomen, *modified* sit-ups are best: Lie on the floor with knees bent and feet flat on the floor, about hip-width apart. Gently clasp hands behind the head or extend straight forward past the knees. Curl up your spine until you can feel the contraction in your abdominal muscles, then slightly relax. Repeat as many times as you can; try to begin with at least a dozen.

Note: When doing sit-ups, do not raise more than your upper back off the floor; more may hurt the back and is of questionable benefit to the abdomen. Just be sure that you are moving right at the point of tension. Increase the number of repetitions as your abdominals become stronger.

Some video workout tapes include excellent all-over stretching routines, but contain a mere minute or two of aerobics. Some who find it convenient to exercise indoors will switch off the tape at this point, do an extra twenty to thirty minutes of jogging in place, then switch back on the tape to finish. (A rebounder will help prevent joint injuries when working out this way indoors.)

The very thought of exercise may be nightmarish if your schedule is already overburdened. It may take a little while, but once you begin to experience the benefits of regular exercise, you will crave it. Perhaps you will change your priorities a little, even give up a few things that no longer seem as essential as exercise.

One university professor who looks twenty years younger than his actual age bought a house close enough to the university where he teaches that he would be able to walk or bicycle to work. For this vigorous man, the optimum distance from work is three miles!

One woman with a beautiful home noticed with dismay the first signs of the shapelessness that can accompany middle age. Now when she sets out for her brisk afternoon walk, she sometimes feels a slight pull to stay inside and make the house perfect and shining. Then she imagines herself ten years from now, in a flabby body and a perfect house—and decides she would rather have a slightly cluttered house.

Some people assuage their guilt feelings over "wasting time" by combining walking with socializing. Others walk alone and claim they get some of their most productive thinking done during their walks.

For people with children, it will help to involve the entire family. We have several friends who go on long biking trips with their young children strapped in special carriers made for kids.

Some people like the structure that is provided by a good gym, and the expert help given by fitness instructors. Others prefer the simple freedom of stepping out into their neighborhood for a walk or a run.

One tremendous motivational element is that the physical benefits of exercise never seem to stop. After six months of working out, you may take pride in your "peak" condition—but make a few adjustments in your routine or length of workout, or try a different sport, and you will find new and wonderful things happening to your body! Changing even one of the three components of a physical workout—intensity, frequency (times per week), and duration (length of workout)—will increase fitness.

.WORKING THE. PROGRAM

One morning Jan was working with a woman who told her she had run seven miles before she came in to work. Jan stopped what she was doing and looked at her. The woman was lean and graceful, she moved easily, and she didn't look tired. "How do you do it?" Jan whispered.

"You have to start the way a child plays," she said. "The child never does the same thing for a long time. The child runs, walks, stops, turns around, skips. Just move, walk and run, and if something hurts, stop."

Jan decided to try this principle the next time she took her daughters swimming. She stayed in the water a long time. She swam a few laps till her lungs began to burn, then she paddled and floated about. She raced her daughter across the pool, then she paddled and floated about. Day by day she found that she grew in strength, until she could swim longer distances. Eventually she was easily swimming a mile at a time.

The idea is to push yourself a little—just enough so that you can feel your heart pound and breathing becomes a little difficult. What you are doing is making your exertion directly proportional to your own body's condition, not to the condition of someone else's body, or to the numbers on a chart. Having included a walking chart in this chapter, obviously we have nothing against charts—*except* when they discourage people from beginning an exercise program. If the chart is helpful to you, make use of it; if not, ignore it! The point is that whatever taxes your body moderately is what you should be doing. If it causes real pain, or is painfully arduous, please don't give up—just *let* up a little.

Now—once you have tasted the joys of physical activity with this playful approach, you will want to get serious. Remember, sustained activity is your goal, for it is only this kind of activity that will condition your heart and burn lots of calories. You may want to follow a chart to help with your progress, perhaps the walking chart in this book, or one of Dr. Ken Cooper's charts for other activities (see list of books below).

It will help to be a little compulsive about your exercise at first. Determine if you will work out four, five, or six times a week, and make yourself do it. After several months of regular exercise, you will anticipate your exercise session as one of the high points of your day.

As with all other endeavors, your thoughts and attitudes will greatly influence your success. It's helpful to read articles and books that will encourage you and give you information. Following is a list of books that we think are particularly helpful.

A good all-around exercise book for those who are not advanced athletes is *If It Hurts, Don't Do It: An Exciting New Program for Pain-Free, Injury-Free, Life-long Fitness,* by Peter and Lorna Francis (Prima Publishing and Communication, 1988). All books on exercise by Dr. Kenneth Cooper (the "inventor" of aerobics!) are motivating and filled with health information. You may want to start with *The New Aerobics* (M. Evans and Co., 1970), or *The Aerobics Program for Total Well-Being* (M. Evans and Co., 1982).

Walking Program

Under 30 Years of Age

Week	Distance (Miles)	Time (Min.)	Freq./ Week	Fitness Maintenance
1–2	1	14	5	At the completion of your
3–5	1.5	21	5	program, you can maintain
6–8	2	28	5	your fitness by walking 3
9–12	2.5	35	5	miles in 42 minutes 5 times a
13–16	3	42	5	week.

30–39 Years of Age

Week	Distance (Miles)	Time (Min.)	Freq./ Week	Fitness Maintenance
1–2	1	15	5	At the completion of your
3–5	1.5	22	5	program, you can maintain
6–9	2	29	5	your fitness by walking 3
10–13	2.5	36	5	miles in 43 minutes 5 times a
14–16	3	43	5	week.

40–49 Years of Age

Week	Distance (Miles)	Time (Min.)	Freq./ Week	Fitness Maintenance
1–3	1	16	5	At the completion of your
4–6	1.5	23	5	program, you can maintain
7–10	2	30	5	your fitness by walking 3
11–14	2.5	37	5	miles in 44 minutes 5 times a
15–16	3	44	5	week.

Ages 50 and Over

Week	Distance (Miles)	Time (Min.)	Freq./ Week	Fitness Maintenance
1–3	1	17	5	At the completion of your
4–6	1.5	24	5	program, you can maintain
7–10	2	31	5	your fitness by walking 3
11–15	2.5	38	5	miles in 45 minutes 5 times a
16	3	45	5	week.

· S U M M A R Y ·

1. Regular exercise has been thought to reduce the risk of many deadly diseases, including diabetes, osteoporosis, cancer (by control-

ling weight), and diseases of the heart and blood vessels; it also helps to control cholesterol levels.

2. Exercise may be the single most important factor in helping to maintain a pleasing and youthful appearance.

3. Exercise relieves stress without drugs, and is a natural mood-lifter.

4. For most people exercise is *the key* to weight control.

5. For exercise to be effective, it must be sustained, and performed a minimum of three times a week, and preferably four or five (even six) times a week.

• This Week's Guide to Success •

Find a partner and make a pact.
Agree that you will walk together five times this week. Set up a time to meet each day and stick to it without fail. If you can't find a partner, join a gym or, at the very least, enlist the support of a friend or family member.

Use the walking chart and try to complete the distance in the time specified for your age group.
Determine a pleasant route, measuring the distance in your car or using a pedometer.

At the end of the week, discuss your exercise plan with your partner, or with a friend or family member.
Will you continue walking, using the walking chart? Would you like to try another form of exercise?

Above all, don't be stopped permanently by difficulties in making exercise a part of your life.
Use whatever help you can—friends, walking groups, videos, exercise classes, biking clubs, etc.

7

· *Principle No. 7* ·

Program Your Mind for Success

It is a law of the mind that it will narrow or expand to the dimensions of the things with which it becomes familiar.
—Ellen G. White

Chris writes:
Is there anything we can do to fight the influences that want to form us into unthinking overweight consumers? It's a battle that *can* be won, day by day. We can take action and *choose the forces* that we want to form our minds; we can say no to the interests that seem to want to keep us fat, malleable, and numbed; and we can help ourselves so we may become slim, strong mentally and physically— and in charge of our own lives.

In the early 1970s my life was governed by physical disease, emotional turmoil, and spiritual defeat. After the birth of my second child I began to take on a chunky appearance due to a dietary life-style I had been comfortable with since I was a child. Every morning I performed the ritual of sitting exhausted on the edge of my bed, waiting to see if I would muster the strength to rise or lie down in defeat. If I found the strength to get up, by midmorning I needed to revive my dissipating energy with a quick "pick-me-up" of my favorite junk foods—only to see midafternoon arrive with an energy crisis that found me simply going through the necessary motions for the rest of the day. My daily resources consisted of little or no breakfast, a fattening lunch with loads of snacks along the way, and an instant dinner of "foodless" convenience foods. In an effort to boost my energy I also consumed a steady diet of television, radio, movies, and adver-

176

tisements—all promising to make me feel "good all over!" But this program of mind manipulation left me depleted, in a constant state of exhaustion—physical, mental, and spiritual. With the added stresses of being a professional career person, wife, mother, and housekeeper, I had become a spendthrift of my life's vital forces. My body began to serve notice in the form of chronic degenerative diseases: kidney disease, severe degenerative arthritis, and ulcerative colitis.

Was this all there was to life? It was a half-baked existence, crumbling under continual stress and crippling diseases!

It was at this critical point in my life that I allowed myself to learn how health is a blending of the physical, mental, and spiritual well-being of the person.

In his 1853 book, *Esoteric Anthropology,* Dr. T. L. Nichols wrote:

When a man is perfect in his own nature, body, and soul, perfect in their harmonious adaptations and action, and living in perfect harmony with nature, with his fellow man, and with God, he may be said to be in a state of health!

More beautifully, Walt Whitman wrote of health:

In that condition the whole body is elevated to a state by others unknown—inwardly and outwardly illuminated, purified, made solid, strong, yet buoyant. A singular charm, more than beauty, flickers out of and over the face—a curious transparency beams in the eyes, both in the iris and the white—the temper partakes also. . . . The play of the body in motion takes a previously unknown grace. Merely to move is then a happiness, a pleasure—to breathe, to see, is also. All the beforehand gratifications, drink, spirits, coffee, grease, stimulants, mixtures, late hours, luxuries, deeds of the night, seem as vexatious dreams, and now the awakening;—many fall into their natural places, wholesome, conveying diviner joys.

We are made of body, mind, and spirit, and any meaningful attempt at health maintenance must be directed to all dimensions of our being. But how do you use the resources of the whole person to attain health for the whole person?

As a Seventh-Day Adventist, I believe that what we physically put into our bodies has a tremendous impact on how we act and feel. Faulty nutrition habits can have a direct impact on one's personality and behavior!

But as important as nutrition is, simply handing someone a diet to follow is not the answer. Dr. Theodore Van Itallie, the famed nutritionist at Columbia University Medical School, suggests: "You don't change the individual by changing his diet; you change his diet by changing him."

It was during the dark crisis in my own life that I learned that this idea must become a reality. The change must begin with me! But how to go about it? I appeared to be helplessly locked into behaviors that were draining my life forces. What was I to do?

In my reading I discovered a critically important principle, which must be understood when one becomes serious about using the resources of the mind to achieve success. *We become what we think about.* Everything we are presently or will become is partly the fruit of the content of our minds. Consequently, anything we do to improve the quality of our thinking can have a positive and tangible reflection in our lives.

The mind was created with the remarkable ability to conform to sensory input. Sounds, sights, and sensations are conveyed from the outside world through a network of more than 12 billion brain cells. Our ears, eyes, and fingers gather the raw data, and the information is fed into the memory base of the brain. From this storehouse of data, thoughts are drawn and commands are given to each organ to perform its task. Whether we achieve our goals is dependent upon our willingness not only to make choices based on this data, but to *choose positive sights and sounds* to be transported into the brain.

If we *don't* choose them—they will be chosen for us!

In his book *As a Man Thinketh,* the nineteenth-century Englishman James Allen wrote, "The mind is like a garden and like a garden either weeds or flowers will grow, but if you do not deliberately, consciously, purposely plant flowers; weeds will grow." Unless we consciously cultivate positive, healthy thoughts consistent with our ideals and objectives in life, the weeds of self-defeat and self-destruction will grow profusely. If we want to have positive experiences, we must consciously focus on positive thought patterns.

Here we come to another vital mental law—the law of repetition. Every ideal, belief, value, and attitude is either a positive or negative thought habit pattern. If you want to stop having negative thoughts, you must repeat positive thought habits.

We live in a time where the messages broadcast by hi-tech media are the most powerful influences in the lives of many of us. They are what we "behold" every day, and they are repeated again and again. For people in other times, the battle was against ignorance and superstition; for many of us today, the battle is against intrusive messages that come over the airwaves or assault our senses in print.

Madison Avenue has "sold" us an obese life-style. Biochemist Paul A. Stitt, in the introduction to his book *Fighting the Food Giants,* states:

Without your knowledge or consent, they control what you eat, when you eat, how much you eat, even the way you think of food.

We are programmed to desire the very foods that make us fat. And as long as this software of high-calorie trash continues to filter through our minds, we will continue to crash-diet and manage the fat for a season only to be compelled by our life-style to go back to old, faulty habit patterns. Can we resist this conditioning? Every television program, every radio broadcast, every billboard and poster message, every newspaper, book, and magazine—all aim their arsenal of marketing strategy at the great citadel of the brain, the control center of decision and action. They storm the bastions of the mind through the senses, as Al Ries, a marketing consultant, explains in his book *Positioning: The Battle for Your Mind:*

Each day, thousands of advertising messages compete for a share of the prospect's mind. And make no mistake about it, the mind is the battleground. Between 6 inches of gray matter is where the advertising war takes place. And the battle is rough with no holds barred and no quarter given.

Day by day, the battle is fought for the attention, the brain cells, the memory, the subconscious, and the will.

The daily use of your senses establishes who you are and will ultimately determine your life's destiny. The senses serve as pathways into your thought processes and will determine how you think, feel, and, hence, act.

Psychologist Leonard Berkowitz reported in a 1964 *Scientific American* article that depiction of violent behavior on the screen and stage stimulated aggressive, combative behavior. His conclusions are drawn from research conducted by him and other scientists. In a controlled study of male hospital attendants in a Canadian hospital and in other studies of young children, he perceived a sizable increase in hostility in individuals subjected to film violence. Male hospital attendants who viewed a filmed knife fight were harsh in punishing patients in comparison to attendants who had not seen the film. Preschool children who were exposed to adult film violence or cartoons displaying violence imitated the violent behavior they observed. Researchers at the University of North Carolina Child Development Center discovered that nursery school children exposed to film violence were more combative than their friends, "some even tripling their violent acts, kicking, choking, hitting, pushing." What you see—and hear—can have an impact on your life to the degree that your behavior can be changed!

It's impossible to renew our ideals and objectives while negative information is continually received through the senses. We think about that which we taste, see, hear, touch, and smell. These senses serve as gateways into our thought processes—they are the sources of thought patterns. Whatever enters the mind through these channels will ultimately express itself in words and behavior.

No one can completely block out all unwanted messages—try driving down the highway without noticing the billboards!—but look at all advertising with a jaundiced eye. What are they trying to sell you? Is it something that will help you achieve your goals, become who *you* want to be? Don't allow yourself to be fooled by clever pitches that try to exploit your desire for health and well-being—you can pay dearly for promises that can't be delivered!

Just as you take care to put nutritious food in your body, take care to give your mind food for inspiration. No one can dictate to you what this material will be—each individual's program will be different. But the search for the right stimuli is a worthwhile search.

Set aside a special time in the morning for centering your mind. Thirty minutes is a good block of time for inspirational reading and thought. We call it the Golden Thirty. Your life may dictate that you practice the Golden Thirty (or the Golden Fifteen!) in the evening or some other time of day. But the morning is ideal: Your mind is rested, there are fewer distractions, and it is a good time to prepare for the day. If you are religious, talk to God. Read something that will inspire you.

As a Seventh-Day Adventist I have found strength and guidance through reading the Bible and the writings of Ellen G. White and other inspirational authors. The challenge is to find inspirational material to put into your mind that will make you feel strong and positive—not weak, hostile, or depressed. Life is full of stress and messages we cannot control, and it would not be practical or desirable to insulate ourselves from these things entirely. But we *can* give ourselves thirty minutes to fortify ourselves for the rest of the day. Try to do it every day.

Another practice that helps strengthen the mind is the repetition of statements known as affirmations. Affirmations are positive, personal present-tense statements that can help you achieve your goals. Do you want to lose weight? Listen to the difference in the following statements. "I've got to lose weight. I've got to lose weight . . ." Now repeat the following statement several times: "I am slim and strong. I am slim and strong . . ."

Which statement feels best to you? Which one do you think would help you acquire the strength to achieve your potential? Find some affirmations that feel good to you and repeat them to yourself throughout the day. Affirmations are natural mood-lifters that often work very quickly to strengthen your mind and to help you feel good about yourself.

My practical health education consisted of learning how to use the first six principles in this book. But it was in applying the principles in the current chapter that I found the staying power for success. No longer am I battling the extra pounds that typify a life-style out of control. At the age of forty-two, I have a greater level of energy and vitality than I had at twenty-two. No longer am I fighting kidney disease, ulcerative colitis, and severe degenerative arthritis. Those are conditions long overcome by the simple realization that the living body must have positive life-enhancing food—physically, mentally, and spiritually.

. W O R K I N G T H E .
P R O G R A M

Jan writes:

The "whole person" concept that Seventh-Day Adventists embrace is so sensible and seems so right that it is a wonder that we sometimes think we can achieve perfect health by paying attention to just one or two aspects of our beings. Everything works together—and neglecting one aspect of our existence makes it more difficult to achieve success in the others.

Chris's experience with overcoming disabling diseases through a combination of sound nutrition and mental conditioning may seem incredible to some. In fact, there is now evidence that suggests that a dietary regime such as the one Chris followed can indeed be helpful in fighting disease. In 1984 researchers at Johns Hopkins Medical Center used a low-protein, high-complex-carbohydrate diet with no meat to stop the progression of kidney disease in twenty-four patients. Dr. Mackenzie Walser stated, "Dietary treatment promises to reduce the needs for dialysis considerably." Chris completely avoided meat and cheese when she began her new diet; these are foods that are often implicated in the development of ulcerative colitis. A low–animal protein diet has also been shown to be of benefit to those suffering from arthritis.

When you add to this diet a program of mental conditioning designed to make you cheerful, positive, and strong—disease may not have a chance! Several popular books in recent years have chronicled the success that some have had by using mental and spiritual techniques to combat disease.

The longer lives of many Seventh-Day Adventists result from a number of things: their avoidance of smoking and drinking, their choice of healthful foods, their emphasis on exercise and on family time together—and also some practices that, among other things, are believed to help in coping with stress.

The observance of the Sabbath, which falls on Saturday for Seventh-Day Adventists, means many things to Chris—among them, she told me, it is a remarkable stress-reliever that she and her family "couldn't do without." On this day they do no work—no cooking, no housework—and they spend the day in rest, in the form of worship, reading, fellowship with family and friends, and service to others.

"That would *increase* my stress!" I told Chris. "I'd be too busy thinking about all the things I had to do!"

"I don't think so," she replied. "The other six days of the week we have been working hard, many of us working long hours. This is a day during which we set aside our cares, recover from the stresses of the week—the next day we are ready to begin with renewed strength!"

Many of us push ourselves, working to exhaustion, with work and worries constantly on our minds. When we take a break, it may be to do something that does not really help us, or that makes us feel better for just a short while (such as gorging on fattening foods or watching a silly television program). Few people will observe the Sabbath as the Adventists do. But perhaps we can make a commitment to ourselves to put our work aside at regular intervals and to find things that will refresh our souls at those times.

Chris's recommendation that we block out commercial messages and degrading messages from our consciousness is intriguing, especially interesting in these times when censorship is a hot political issue. The interesting thing is that Adventists on the whole *do not believe in external censorship*. This is because as a group they believe strongly in the separation of church and state—that personal beliefs, no matter how deeply held, should not be enforced by the government. Thus, the "censorship" Chris speaks of is a matter of *personal choice,* made by the *individual*. Those of us who feel strongly about our First Amendment rights believe that no one has the right to tell us what we may or may not listen to or look at. But does this mean we must passively take in whatever images or messages are beamed our way—even if those messages cause us to feel bad?

The trick is learning what it is you want to fill your mind with and what it is you want to block out as far as is possible. You learn these things through experience, through reading, through thinking, and through listening to those you trust.

As for the affirmations—they really work! None of the principles we present in this book are magic—but if anything can *feel* like magic, it is a well-used affirmation.

The most successful affirmations are those that counter a negative thought that may often run through your mind. Often these negative thoughts are present without our full awareness of them. But they are powerful. If you can "catch" a negative thought pattern and convert it into a positive, present-tense statement that you repeat *many times,* you will be surprised to discover how much you can accomplish *and* how much happier you will feel.

For example, at the bottom of your uneasy feelings about a new diet may be the thought: "I am no good at staying on diets." Change this thought to: "It is easy for me to eat the right amounts of healthful foods"—and see how much easier it *does* become!

• S U M M A R Y •

1. Nutrition habits can have a direct impact on your personality and behavior.

2. Any successful attempt at maintaining health must be directed to the entire being, including body, mind, and spirit (the "whole person" concept).

3. The content of our minds so influences the type of person we are that it may be said: *We become what we think about.* Successful goal achievement is dependent on the willingness of an individual not only to make choices based on the information his brain receives, but to *choose positive sights and sounds* to be transported into the brain.

4. The positive information we choose to put into our minds should be repeated often, renewed daily. Thirty minutes in the morning for inspiration and meditation is ideal.

5. Affirmations are positive, present-tense statements that, when repeated often, will help you achieve your potential and provide you with a natural lift in mood.

• This Week's Guide to Success •

FOR SPIRITUAL DEVELOPMENT

Fortification: Take advantage of the early morning time, the Golden Thirty, to read positive inspirational material to fortify your mind and spirit against the inevitable invasion of negative information.

Communion: Converse with God, expressing intimately your feelings, hopes, and desires. If you are not religious, place your mind on positive, life-enhancing things that are important to you.

Reflection: Try to reserve a quiet time at the close of each day for reflection and examination of your experiences.

FOR MENTAL DEVELOPMENT

Affirmation: Each day make positive, present-tense, personal assertive statements that say *yes* to your potential:

I am slender.
I eat foods that make me healthy.
I can do all things through Christ which strengtheneth me.
　(Phillippians 4:13).
I grow stronger in body, mind, and spirit.

Visualization: Form a clear, concise mental picture of who you want to be and retain that picture very clearly in your mind. Throughout the day, visualize yourself slim and trim, eating healthy foods, making positive choices.

FOR PHYSICAL DEVELOPMENT

Nutrition: Follow the Menu Planner. Consume six to eight glasses of water daily.

Exercise: Plan to incorporate an aerobic form of exercise into your day at least three times weekly, for thirty to sixty minutes. For serious weight loss, increase this to five times weekly.

Sensory experience: Avoid as much as possible negative sensory input. Everything that traverses the threshold of our minds affects our thinking and changes us. Choose positive, life-enhancing experiences for the senses to enjoy. This is the key to a new you.

8

Making It Easy

In this chapter we will explore some ideas that can make it easier to become slim and healthy. Please remember this: The whole program gets *easier* and *easier* as you begin to feel better and have more energy.

The Restaurant Plan

The Restaurant Plan is an idea that is especially good for working people, single people, and for those who have *no time to cook*. It takes the least amount of time, and only requires being able to get to a good health food restaurant at lunchtime.

If you live or work near a Seventh-Day Adventist restaurant, then you have it made! In answer to Ellen G. White's call, Seventh-Day Adventists established cooking schools and restaurants throughout the world. If there isn't one in your town, there may be another kind of restaurant that emphasizes fresh, healthful foods. Quite often vegetarian restaurants are the very best at coming up with tasty, high-protein dishes that use fresh vegetables, whole grains, and legumes. However, there are also restaurants that are not strictly vegetarian that may serve your needs.

Here's how the plan works. Your shopping list will be a short one, of milk, whole-grain cereal, bread, peanut butter, and fruit. This will give you everything you need for breakfast, as outlined in the Menu Planner.

At lunchtime you will eat a restaurant meal that conforms as closely as possible to the guidelines in the Menu Planner. Please pay special attention to the vegetables, including one green leafy vegetable and at least one raw vegetable or salad, if possible.

186

Now, when you get home after work—there is no cooking to do! If you are eating the optional light supper, you simply eat a plateful of fruit.

It's easy!

Dinner at Breakfast Time

Eating dinner at breakfast time is a way of working the plan that is especially good for families whose life is centered around work and family. It is also good for those who must carry lunches to work or school. Eat dinner in the morning (by "dinner" we mean a substantial protein-and-vegetable meal), and pack simple lunches of sandwiches and fruit.

This plan is a great boon for the primary meal-preparer of the family, for late afternoon is often the low time of the day. It eliminates that deadly hour when an exhausted parent is trying to prepare dinner, ignoring his or her own hunger pangs while demanding children complain and fight.

If a substantial, nutritious dinner has been eaten early in the morning, the parent may relax his or her vigilance for the rest of the day, for the children have already "gotten their vegetables." If the children are hungry after school or in the evening—let them get their own! Keep granola, fruit, bread, and leftovers in the kitchen for them. There are better things to do after a hard day's work than to spend time cooking and cleaning up a big dinner. How about relaxing, exercising, or spending time with family and friends?

There are, of course, potential problems with serving dinner early in the morning. It may be necessary to get up earlier. But this need not be an insurmountable problem if you have made preparations beforehand. If you have soups and casseroles in the freezer you can take them out the night before and heat them up in the morning. The crockpot is also a big help in preparing food that is ready to eat in the morning.

Another potential problem is in getting the family used to a new routine. It may be best at first with children not to make drastic changes in the *type* of food you serve them. It is a big enough adjustment to eat dinner in the morning. Your children may laugh when they wake up to the smell of spaghetti or pizza—but they may like it! They will feel good, have more energy at school, and will like the fact that their parents have more time for them in the evening. A child made miserable by a weight problem will be delighted to find that his or her weight is more easily controlled when he or she eats a large breakfast (encourage the child to eat *lightly* in the afternoon and evening).

Another problem may be the thorny "social" one. See Chapter 5 for some ideas on this subject. In fact, among working people there is a decided trend toward a healthier life-style, and that includes a greater emphasis on the morning meal.

Setting Up the Kitchen

If you like to cook, you may already know how helpful it is to have your kitchen really well organized. A cook who makes an effort to set up the kitchen intelligently will find that cooking takes much less time than when done in a haphazard manner.

Of course, every style of cooking calls for its own particular type of organization. The Seventh-Day Adventist style may be a little different from any you have tried before. Once you become familiar with it, however, you will find that it falls on the easy end of the spectrum. Like other cooking styles, it has its own set of customary seasonings and ingredients, and once the basics are acquired and organized, it is quite easy to make any recipe in this book—and to create your own.

In the spirit of simplicity, we have not overwhelmed you with dozens of recipes; we have simply selected the best. You may wish to master only a few of the more involved dishes to serve on special occasions; for everyday meals, cook simply, with fresh and simple ingredients.

Following are some ideas on how to organize your kitchen. Your own plan will vary depending on your kitchen and your own cooking needs.

You may already own a variety of baking dishes that will serve for the recipes in this book. If you plan on buying more, you should know that the most common sizes of pans used in the recipes in this book are 8 x 8 inches, 11½ x 8 inches, and 13 x 9 inches. Buy glass baking dishes—if you can find them with snap-on plastic covers for storage, so much the better. If you love to make pies, you probably want to buy a nice deep pie plate or two, in the 9-inch size.

Because it is unlikely (and even undesirable) that your family will

give up their accustomed foods all at once, you may begin by desig-
nating one cabinet in your kitchen as your "healthful foods" cooking
cabinet. Here you will keep most of the special ingredients and seasonings that are called for in the recipes in this book. On the counter
beneath this cabinet you might place your blender—*the* most important appliance. Keep it close to the sink so that it can easily be
cleaned by half filling with warm water and a squirt of dishwashing
liquid, blended to a froth, then rinsed out under the tap.

Inside the cooking cabinet are seasonings arranged on two lazy
Susans on the bottom shelf. These are the pleasing and diges-
tible seasonings that the Seventh-Day Adventists use, such as
ground coriander, sweet basil, and thyme. (A more complete list of
these seasonings is found in Chapter 9.) On the left-hand side
are the seasonings that begin with letters in the first half of the
alphabet; the rest are placed on the right. (Well, yes, this is a bit
compulsive. But it *does* make it easier to quickly find the right
ingredients!)

Also in this cabinet are canned goods such as pimientos, crushed
unsweetened pineapple, olives, etc. By now you know that we emphasize the use of fresh ingredients when possible, but there are a few
healthful and necessary exceptions.

On the shelf above are other basic ingredients: Bakon seasoning, a
canister of brewer's yeast flakes, a bottle of lecithin, soy sauce, Soyagen, and other ingredients that you will find described in Chapter
9. On the top shelf you may wish to keep the mixing bowls and baking
dishes that you use most often.

Measuring cups and spoons should be close at hand, perhaps the
cups on the same shelf as the seasonings and the spoons in a drawer
below.

Next to the blender you might place your crockpot. While you may
not use it as often as the blender, it is convenient to have it where
you can easily fill it with beans and seasonings and other ingredients
for overnight cooking.

If you have lots of storage space, and if you prefer a "clean-counter
kitchen," you may keep most of your ingredients in cabinets. Some
people, however, prefer to line up on their counters glass containers
filled with staple ingredients: sunflower seeds, millet, coconut,
honey, sesame seeds, etc. These may be simply containers that have
held other foods and juices, or you may buy decorative canisters for
this purpose.

If you have room to store things and find you often run out of a particular ingredient, it is helpful to buy it in large quantities. Beans, rice, and oatmeal are especially convenient to have on hand.

On a hook to the right of the sink you may wish to permanently hang a large colander—used for draining pasta, or course, but also necessary for rinsing those ubiquitous cashews! Keeping often-used utensils like this one in plain sight right at hand can really save time. In the same spirit, you may wish to keep your collapsible steamer on a hook above the stove or on a counter nearby.

A chopping board and several sharp knives should also be at hand. If you have a food processor, it can substitute for much of the knife work.

Now for the refrigerator. As you move toward health, your refrigerator will contain more juices and fresh vegetables and fruits. As suggested in Chapter 2, it is good to devote substantial space to the fresh produce you have so carefully selected; perhaps one drawer for fruit, one for vegetables, and maybe an entire shelf for half-prepared or cut-up fruits and vegetables.

In the freezer go plenty of bananas, those very ripe ones that you have peeled and wrapped in plastic wrap in order to use them for drinks and desserts. Also in the freezer are frozen juice concentrates and already-prepared portions of beans and casseroles.

A kitchen such as this one provides everything you need to do some fantastic healthful cooking.

A New Way to Cook, One Step at a Time

You may not want to do a major overhaul of your kitchen all at once. You may be afraid that all those new ingredients will strain your budget beyond repair. Let's face it—a radical change in cooking style can be very expensive if you buy a whole collection of new ingredients all at once, determined to make special recipes every day. It's sad when this happens, for the new cook often gets the idea that healthful cooking is always expensive! There are ways to keep costs down, and a very important way is to concentrate on beans and grains such as rice for everyday cooking. Good health food store personnel can also give you advice on cooking with economy, and point out thrifty ways of buying ingredients.

If you want to adopt this new cooking style slowly, we suggest you begin with the recipe for Pimiento Cashew Cheese (page 135). A spoonful of this sauce is great on steamed or raw vegetables, beans, grains—in fact, it is hard to think of a nonsweet food that it is *not* good on! It is a common ingredient in many of the entrée recipes in this book. You may find it helpful to keep a copy of the recipe pinned to the inside of your "health cabinet" door, and for convenience in preparing the fresh lemon juice, you may want to keep a lemon juicer on a hook inside the cabinet. With a bag of lemons in the refrigerator and all the other ingredients in or below the cabinet, you have every- thing you need to make this flavorful sauce.

With the addition of soy sauce and optional ground coriander, you also have everything you need to make Southern-Style Gravy (page 141). This is another recipe you may wish to copy and tack to the inside of the cabinet door. It's great on potatoes and is also a basic ingredient in some of the entrée recipes.

Your next project may be a big batch of beans simmered on the stove or in the crockpot, some to be eaten at once, some to be frozen for later.

Try the Garden Patch Potato Stack (page 73) and Haystacks (page 117). These recipes will give you a good idea of what everyday Adven- tist cooking is all about. These dishes provide everything you need for a nutritious, flavorful meal, and they feature a "stacking tech- nique" that you can use to create other easy meals. It will quickly become obvious to you that you can easily create your own dishes, using the vegetables that you happen to have on hand. Try using pasta or rice for the first layer of your layered dishes.

A person who lives alone may want to freeze part of a casserole for future meals and keep the rest in the refrigerator for immediate consumption.

Raw vegetables are important in maintaining health and ideal weight, and they also contribute to simplicity in food preparation. Make a casserole, soup, or entrée; serve it with bread and a big platter of raw vegetables; and you have a very satisfying meal.

The World Is Making It Easier

People have become more concerned about their health. At the same time, health care has become terrifyingly expensive. Many have be- come convinced that *prevention* of disease, aided by a plan such as the one in this book, is the surest and least expensive way to stay healthy. What this means is that our society will gradually become one in which it is easier to follow a healthy way of life.

Some people will want to spend more time preparing food for their families once they become convinced how important it is. Some will find their energies channeled in other directions, but nevertheless will want to eat delicious, healthful food and to provide it for their families. Our hope is that some of those who find fulfillment in preparing food will harness that impulse and put it to work. Maybe they'll begin to rethink their careers, finding creative satisfaction in providing health-giving food, seeking out ways to live more healthy lives and helping others to follow. We need people who will give careful attention to the preparation of life-sustaining food, and we need to cultivate respect for those who provide this service.

Is eating carefully prepared foods more expensive than subsisting on fast, greasy foods? It is certainly *less* expensive than the costs of hospitalization and major surgery that are becoming a terrible burden on individuals and on the public!

Making health feasible is not simply a matter of appliances and schedules; it is also facilitated by the thoughts and efforts of other people, a growing awareness of what is good in our society, a kind of spirit of the age. Doctors who become aware of the importance of diet and exercise can teach their patients the importance of these things; food-service workers can put their efforts into preparing fresh, delicious foods for consumers; agriculturists can develop ways of producing fresh, pesticide-free food that all can afford; and consumers can demand this kind of food. It's going to take a lot of people working together.

The good news? It's already beginning to happen.

• SUMMARY •

1. The easiest way to work this plan is to eat a simple breakfast of cereal, bread, and fruit, then eat your substantial meal at lunchtime at a healthy foods restaurant. The evening meal, if eaten, will be a plate of fruit.

2. Some people will find it most expedient to serve the substantial vegetable meal ("dinner") at breakfast time, and to carry a lunch of sandwiches and fruit.

3. Taking time to organize the kitchen according to your cooking needs will save time in the long run and will help make your cooking chores pleasurable rather than frustrating.

4. Most people will do better adopting healthier eating habits if they make changes *gradually*.

5. Some of the difficulties in trying to follow a healthy way of life will be alleviated as more and more people become aware of the physical, mental, and financial rewards that come from preventive health practices.

9

Natural Foods Shopping Guide

You may choose to follow the Menu Planner very simply, using the more familiar kinds of whole grains, nuts, beans, and fresh produce; or you may find pleasure in experimenting with creative combinations of foods, including some of the lesser-known but delicious varieties that we list in this chapter.

To help you begin stocking up for your new cuisine, we're giving you a shopping list and a little bit of supermarket savvy. Please don't feel you must purchase all of the items mentioned in order to begin the program. This list is provided to make you aware of the wide range of foods that are available to make your diet more enjoyable and interesting.

It's best to move into the program gradually, replacing nutrient-depleted foods with more healthful substitutes. Buy small amounts until you've discovered which products you like. Once your kitchen is completely stocked with healthful, life-giving foods, you will find that eating a plant-based diet is not only slenderizing and appetizing, but economical!

Reading Labels

It is important to get in the habit of reading labels carefully. Please be aware that words such as "natural," "pure," or "whole" have become overused—and often misused—in the world of commercial foods. Manufacturers often stamp these words on products that actually may have no special health-giving value. Another deceptive manufacturer's practice is to place on the packaging in bold letters phrases such as "no added sugar," "no preservatives," "no cholesterol," or "low fat." Such phrases do not convey what exactly the product contains and generally are no validation of its healthfulness.

A corn oil label that reads "cholesterol-free" simply means that that brand of corn oil is just like all other brands of corn oil: Corn oil is a vegetable product and *never* contains cholesterol!

In any event, always read the fine print on the label. The law requires that most food labels list the ingredients in order of predominance. Clearly, food items that tend to increase the risk of disease should be avoided. Sugar, white flour products, solid fat or shortening, and preservatives, if not entirely eliminated, should be kept to a bare minimum. These are empty or refined calories that contribute very little to the body's requirements for vitamins, minerals, essential fats, protein, and fiber.

Sugar. Most sugar is hidden in foods that may appear quite innocent. Sugar is disguised in many ways on labels—as "brown sugar," "sucrose," "dextrose," "maltose," "fructose," "corn syrup," "malt," "molasses," and "honey." Even the more benign sweeteners such as honey, when added to several other *types* of sweetener, can result in a product that is largely sugar!

White flour products. Remember, don't be tricked by the terms "enriched," "restored," or "degerminated"—these words just mean you've been robbed! Foods that may be so labeled include white bread, rice, flour, refined cereals, crackers, pasta, and sweetened bakery goods.

Hard fats. Hard fats are generally described on a packaging label as "animal fat," "lard," "hydrogenated vegetable oils," or "partially hydrogenated oils." Hydrogenation occurs when liquid vegetable oils are hardened with hydrogen, forming chemically saturated fats that do not provide the advantages of the essential polyunsaturated fats.

Preservatives. Preservatives are found in many kinds of foods. Most of their names are hard to pronounce and just as difficult to remember. Even if you can't pronounce or remember the names, just remember that they extend the shelf-life of the product, but not *your* life!

The habit of reading labels will help keep harmful synthetic or engineered foods out of the diet. Limit your food purchases primarily to the products that contain simple, natural ingredients. After all, living people need living food—not clever chemical versions of food designed by manufacturers!

In truth, it is best to spend most of your marketing time with the "greengrocer," and in other sections of the market that carry simple whole foods without complicated labels.

Following is a list of the additives that Adventists believe to be the most harmful. Avoid them if you can!

Alcohol

Baking soda and powder

Caffeine

Gelatin

Lard

Meat and meat fats

Monosodium glutamate (MSG)

Nitrites, nitrates

Potassium bicarbonate

Ripened cheese

Saccharin

Irritating spices (pepper, ginger, cinnamon)

Tea and coffee

Vinegar

And here are the types of junk food that one would do well to avoid: cakes, crackers, pies, and doughnuts; colas, soft drinks, punches, and powdered drinks; frozen pizzas; gelatin and pudding desserts; ice cream and ice milk; beer; vegetable sauces; canned broths; salad dressings.

A Shopping List

Most of the items on this shopping list can be purchased at your supermarket; others you can find at your local health food store or nutrition center. If you can't find something there, ask the manager to order it for you. Managers at health food stores are generally accommodating!

Fruits (Eat generously from this group.)

Apples	Berries	Grapes
Apricots	Cherries	Kiwi
Bananas*	Grapefruit	Lemons*

Mangoes	Papayas	Plums
Melons	Peaches	Pomegranates
Nectarines	Pears	Tangelos
Olives*	Persimmons	Tangerines
Oranges	Pineapple	

Dried Fruits (These are concentrated foods and should be eaten in smaller amounts.)

Apples	Figs	Pears
Apricots	Mangoes	Pineapples
Bananas	Papayas	Prunes
Currants	Peaches	Raisins
Dates*		

Vegetable Fruits (Botanically classified as fruits because they contain seeds, these foods are widely regarded as vegetables. However you think of them, eat generously.)

Avocadoes*	Squash
Cucumbers	Tomatoes
Eggplant	
Peppers (green, red, and yellow)	

Vegetables (Eat generously of these foods.)

Artichokes	Collards	Shallots
Asparagus	Green beans	Snap beans
Beets	Jerusalem artichokes	Snow peas
Bok choy		Spinach
Broccoli	Kale	Sprouts (mung bean, alfalfa, wheat berry, etc.)
Brussels sprouts	Leeks	
Cabbage	Lettuce	
Cauliflower	Mushrooms	Turnip greens
Celery	Mustard greens	
Chard	Peas	

Root Vegetables (Eat generously of these foods.)

Carrots	Potatoes	Sweet potatoes
Daikon radish	Radishes	Turnips
Onions	Rutabagas	Yams
Parsnips		

Grains (Eat three servings daily; each serving should be of a different kind of grain.)

Barley

Breads (whole grain or sprouted):
  Chapatis
  Corn tortillas
  English muffins
  Millet bread
  Pita
  Raisin bread
  Sprouted corn
  Sprouted rye
  Sprouted wheat
  Whole-wheat
  Whole-wheat tortillas

Cereal products (whole grain):
  Cold cereals (fruit-sweetened granola,* Grape-Nuts, Nutri-Grain Wheat, Shredded Wheat)
  Hot cereals (Bearmush, cracked wheat, millet, oatmeal, rice, Wheatena)
  Flakes (barley, oat, rye, triticale, wheat)
  Pasta
  Wild rice

Corn

Cracked wheat (bulgur)

Crackers (whole grain, prepared with yeast, not with baking powder or baking soda):
  Crispbread wafers
  Finn Crisp
  Health Valley crackers
  Hol-Grain Waferets
  Norwegian Ideal whole-grain flatbread
  Ryquita crisp
  Ry-Krisp

Kasha

Millet

Rice:
  Basmati
  Brown

Legumes (Eat several times a week.)

Black beans	Lentils	Pinto beans
Black-eyed peas	Lima beans	Red beans
Garbanzos	Mung beans	Soy beans
Great Northern beans	Navy beans	Split peas (yellow and green)
	Peanuts	
Kidney beans	Pink beans	

Nuts and Seeds (Eat in moderation.)

Almonds	Macadamia nuts	Pumpkin seeds
Brazil nuts	Pecans	Sesame seeds
Cashews*	Pine nuts	Sunflower seeds*
Filberts	Walnuts	

Seed and Nut Butters (Use as spreads on breads, in place of empty-calorie margarine and butter; but spread sparingly.)

Almond	Sesame (tahini)
Cashew	Sunflower
Peanut (in actuality a legume)*	

Dairy Products

If you do use dairy products, select nonfat varieties and use in small quantities. You may use nut milk or soy milk* (Edensoy or Sunsoy) as milk replacements, and soy cheese.

Oils* (Oils are highly concentrated and should be used sparingly.)

Canola	Olive	Sesame
Corn	Safflower	Sunflower

Herbs* (These are pleasing and digestible sweet herbs that are not considered irritating or harmful in any way.)

Bay leaf	Celery seed	Cumin
Caraway seed	Coriander	Dill seed

Herbs (continued)

Dill weed	Paprika	Savory
Fennel	Parsley	Spearmint
Garlic	Peppermint	Sweet basil
Marjoram	Rosemary	Tarragon
Mint	Saffron	Thyme
Oregano	Sage	

Other Seasonings

Bakon Seasoning *

Extracts:
  Almond
  Coconut
  Lemon
  Orange
  Vanilla

Hain's Onion Soup Mix

Hain's Mushroom Soup Mix

Salt substitutes *
  (should contain no
  pepper or sugar)

Soy sauce (Kikkoman
  has a low-sodium brand
  and contains no MSG)

Tamari

Vegetized salt *
  (Vege-Sal, Herbamere)

Miscellaneous Ingredients

Arrowroot *

Carob powder, unsweetened *

Coconut, unsweetened *

Egg substitutes *

Emes Plain Kosher-Jel *

Lecithin *

Nutritional yeast flakes *
(brewer's yeast flakes,
primary yeast flakes,
food yeast flakes)

Soyagen *

Tofu

Herb Teas

Celestial Seasonings   Seelect

Coffee Substitutes (Usually made from barley, figs, chicory, and/or cereal grains.)

Cafix	Pioneer	Roma

Sweeteners

Dates*	Honey*
Date sugar	Sucanat (Raw sugarcane
Juice concentrates*	juice, in granular form)

Following is more detailed information about selected ingredients (those marked with asterisks) on the shopping list:

Arrowroot. Arrowroot is a white powdery substance, made by grinding the root of the arrowroot plant.

It is used as a thickener and a powerful binder, most often in sauces and custards that would normally be thickened by eggs; in roasts and patties; and for thickening creams, gravies, and syrups. What makes it different from flour or cornstarch is that it is not refined to any degree. However, because it is expensive, you may choose to substitute equal amounts of cornstarch in the recipes.

In sauces, syrups, and gravies, be sure to cook arrowroot until it is not only thick but *clear,* or your sauces will have a chalky taste. It also helps to dissolve it in a little cold water before adding it to the rest of the mixture.

Avocado. The avocado is one of "nature's fats" that Adventists view as a healthful and delicious addition to a total vegetarian diet. Used in moderation, it is one of those foods that is going to keep you from feeling deprived. Slice avocados onto salads, and use in guacamole to top baked potatoes and other dishes. But if you still eat a fair amount of animal products, please use avocados in moderation.

Bakon seasoning. Bakon seasoning is a smoked yeast used traditionally by Adventists to add a smoky flavor to food. Health food stores can order Bakon seasoning from Bakon Yeast, Inc., P.O. Box 651, Rhinelander, WI 54501.

Carob. For those who love chocolate, carob is a pleasing, healthful substitute. It is low in fat (2 to 7 percent, as compared with 52 percent fat in chocolate). It is rich in natural sugars, making it unnecessary to add as much sweetener as is required for chocolate. It contains no caffeine. It is a rich source of the following nutrients: vitamin A, calcium, potassium, phosphorus, magnesium, silicon, and iron, and it has its own vitamin B, the vitamin that is necessary to digest simple sugars.

You may buy carob at your health food store in powdered form or in chips—we recommend the chips sweetened with barley or malt. Carob powder should be the kind that is roasted and contains no sugar.

Cashews. The versatile cashew nut has a mild flavor, so it can be incorporated into many kinds of dishes. Because it is soft, it can be blended to a smooth white liquid to make "creamy" sauces.

Nuts are high in fat, so they must be used in moderation—but they contain no cholesterol.

The cashew must be rinsed well before using, as the conditions under which cashews are grown are often less than sanitary.

Be sure to buy raw cashews. The least expensive way is to buy them in *pieces,* in bulk at your health food store.

Coconut. Despite its complete lack of cholesterol, many people are skeptical of coconut—many doctors even place it on the list of "forbidden foods" they give to their patients who are trying to lower their cholesterol. True, its oil is a saturated fat, but it has a lower melting point than hydrogenated fats. We do not use its oil in the recipes in this book, but we use small amounts of the shredded meat of the coconut for flavor and texture.

Seventh-Day Adventists use coconut happily and in moderation, pointing to the lean, healthy island people who live largely on coconuts and who have extremely low rates of heart disease. The saturated fat in coconut does not elevate cholesterol if there is no cholesterol in the diet. Adventists believe that if animal fat is avoided there is no harm in enhancing your diet with judiciously chosen natural plant fats—from coconut, avocado, nuts, etc.

Of course the mainstay of one's diet should be fruits and vegetables —foods with low concentration—but what a boon to be able to use natural plant fats for flavor, especially if you have reduced or eliminated from your diet most visible fats, animal products, and sugar!

Convenience foods. We encourage you to use fresh, whole foods whenever possible. Many "convenience foods"—most packaged baked goods, frozen dinners, packaged mixes—contain ingredients that can either damage your health or, at best, do not sustain it.

Many natural foods are convenient! Think of bananas, grapes, nuts, granola, peanut butter, and dried fruit. Some processed foods such as soy cheese are also healthful and convenient.

There are a few prepared convenience foods that you will find in the recipes in this book: natural onion-soup mix (such as Hain's), natural bottled spaghetti sauce, and vegetable shortening that comes in a spray can.

Dates. We use dates in place of sugar to sweeten cookies, sauces, syrups, and cakes. They are very sweet, but unlike sugar they also contain vitamins, minerals, and fiber. Be sure to check for stray pits before tossing dates into the blender! For those who are wary of date flavor: When you add ground dates to a fruit syrup or other concoction, you do not taste the dates, only their sweetness.

Egg substitutes. There are several things Adventists use in place of eggs for their binding and thickening qualities. One of them, arrowroot, has been mentioned above. Soyagen (soy protein powder) is used in some recipes, such as waffles. The liquid egg substitutes (such as Eggbeaters) that are found frozen in little paper cartons in the freezer section of the grocery store (¼ cup = 1 egg) we have avoided for the most part because they do contain some egg white. However, for some recipes (quiches and some cookies) they are necessary; we have included a small selection of such recipes at the end of the recipes in Chapter 4 for those who want to use them.

Frozen bananas. Frozen bananas are great to have on hand for those times when you want to make refreshing special drinks or frozen fruit desserts. The bananas you freeze should be very ripe, perhaps a little past the point where you would feel comfortable peeling and eating them. A brown-spotted skin means that the natural sugar content of the banana has reached new heights—all that sweetness should not go to waste! You may peel the banana, wrap it in plastic wrap, then place in the freezer.

Frozen bananas allow you to be creative in coming up with special treats. You can put cut-up chunks in the blender with any other fresh or frozen fruit, thinning with a little juice to make a frozen slushy dessert, adding more juice to make a "smoothie."

Frozen juice concentrates. Juice concentrates are another healthful substitute for sugar. But, like dates, though they *are* more healthful than sugar, they are concentrated foods and should be used in moderation.

If a recipe calls for less than a can of juice concentrate and you don't want to make juice out of the rest of the can, store the opened can in a plastic bag in your freezer, ready for the next recipe.

Gelatin. Plain unflavored gelatin may be used in the recipes, but many Adventists use Emes Plain Kosher-Jel, available in the kosher section of your supermarket, from kosher groceries, and from Emes Kosher Products, Lombard, IL 60148.

Granola. Granola is a "convenience food" that, in addition to being eaten as a cold cereal, may be used to make quick fruit crisps and other desserts. Some commercial varieties of granola that are overly sweet and oily have given it a bad name, but there are now wonderful fruit-sweetened varieties available on the market, some with a light and crunchy texture that most people find appealing. They can be found in the nutrition centers of most large grocery stores as well as in health food stores.

And of course you can always make your own special granola (see page 17)!

Honey. Natural unfiltered honey contains small amounts of minerals, protein, B vitamins, and vitamin K, which is known to inhibit tooth decay by halting the formation of acid bacteria in the mouth. (Cane sugar loses its vitamin K in the process of refining.)

As one would expect, the use of honey should be limited. We use it in the occasional dessert because small amounts of honey are not believed to be harmful, while white sugar is best avoided entirely.

Honey is more easily measured if the measuring cup or spoon is oiled first.

Leavenings. You may notice that neither baking soda nor baking powder are used as leavening in the recipes in this book. These ingredients are known to destroy vitamins in the baking process and to leave small amounts of harmful residues that irritate the digestive tract. The yeast used for leavening bread is fine. If you make your own bread, experiment with recipes that use delicious whole grains. Fortunately for those of us who are short on time, many bakeries and most grocery stores now sell wonderful whole-grain breads that are baked with a minimum of fat and salt.

Lecithin. Lecithin is a diglyceride. Its value lies in its ability to disperse or emulsify fat so that it is smoothly distributed throughout the food product. You can see this ability at work when you make the shortening for our flaky pie crust. It is the lecithin that disperses the oil throughout the water and turns it into a white creamy substance.

Lemon juice. Seventh-Day Adventists avoid vinegar because of its acetic acid, which is normally not found in the body, but is often found in the laboratory in a bottle labeled "poison." You will find instead the frequent use of lemon juice gives foods tartness and flavor. Fresh lemon juice is always best.

If a recipe calls for the use of grated lemon peel you may find it most convenient to cut a strip of the yellow part of the peel (none of the white) and place it in the blender with some of the liquid ingredients.

Nutritional yeast flakes. The nutritional yeast used in the recipes in this book is the kind that comes in *flaked* form, not powdered. Ask for it at your health food store. It may be called brewer's yeast, primary yeast, or food yeast flakes—whatever it is called, make sure you buy *flakes*. It contains high-quality protein, B-complex vitamins, iron, phosphorus, and other minerals. Some fortified types contain vitamin B_{12} (important knowledge for those who eat no animal products).

Oil. The use of oil should be kept to a minimum. However, a diet completely without oils, or unsaturated fats, is not recommended except for certain kinds of therapeutic diets. Unsaturated fats are an essential part of the diet, providing energy, working as carriers for the fat-soluble vitamins A, D, E, K, and aiding in the absorption of vitamin D and calcium. Diets devoid of unsaturated fatty acids could lead to unhealthy weight loss and eczematous conditions of the skin. The unsaturated fatty acids provided by nature (in nuts, legumes, grains, and fruits) are the most easily digested. Remember, olive oil keeps the arteries more elastic, canola oil helps to keep the blood from clotting, and other oils such as sunflower, safflower, corn, and sesame can help lower blood cholesterol.

Olives. Avoid green olives—they are loaded with salt. Black olives are fine. Ellen White said it wouldn't hurt you to eat ripe olives at every meal. Indulge!

Pasta. There is a wonderful variety of pasta on the market. Try whole-wheat pasta—but if you don't like it, don't despair. If you're not ready for the "brown look," but want a pasta that is better nutritionally than that made of white flour, try Jerusalem artichoke pasta or soy flour pasta. Even better is lupini (made from lupin seed and wheat) or quinoa pasta. Both are very high in protein and fiber and make a great high-protein meal with vegetables—even though they look white!

Corn pasta is fine nutritionally, but it tends to fall apart during cooking.

Peanut butter. Many commercial peanut butters trumpet the fact that they contain no cholesterol—which is true enough—but they neglect to trumpet the fact that the shortening they contain is hydrogenated, a process that reduces the good, polyunsaturated, essential fatty acids. The best peanut butter is the natural kind, ground from peanuts with sometimes a touch of salt. It is easy to find in any grocery store as well as in health food stores.

This "good" peanut butter often needs to be stirred to disperse the oil throughout. Store it in the refrigerator to keep the oil from separating again. To make it easier to spread or to mix with other ingredients, it can be heated gently until it softens.

Salt. Salt is a blessing as a flavor enhancer. Its use should be minimized, but for most healthy people it need not be eliminated entirely. The current recommendation is to reduce salt intake to one teaspoon of added salt per day, or less. The number one source of salt in the American diet is meat; then refined foods; then *added table salt*. If you confine your salt use to the amounts called for in the recipes in this book, you will be doing fine. Just don't add any more at the table —and remember to eat plenty of raw foods, too.

If you are on a salt-restricted diet, either eliminate salt from the recipes or use a salt substitute. Many salt substitutes contain potassium chloride instead of sodium chloride—these should not be taken without a physician's advice.

You may want to try Vege-Sal. It is a vegetable seasoning salt that doesn't contain any harmful spices.

Seasonings. The seasonings on the shopping list are the "sweet herbs" that do not harm the digestive tract. Adventists avoid irritating condiments and spices (some of which are now suspected of being carcinogenic!).

Those whose palates are accustomed to spicy foods may not at first appreciate more simply seasoned foods. But once you become accustomed to them—and to how good they make you feel!—the "other kind" will not be as appealing. You may have noticed the extensive use of coriander in the recipes. It is an ancient aromatic herb that Adventists use in place of cinnamon or nutmeg, which are thought to be irritants. It has the taste of nutmeg, cinnamon, sage, and a hint of lemon peel. Please be sure to buy the ground *seeds*, not the dried *leaves*, which have a completely different flavor.

Soyagen. This is a commercial soy protein powder that is often used as a binder in place of eggs.

Soy cheese. This is a product made from organic soy milk that simulates the taste and texture of real cheese. It is not aged. The use of ripe, aged cheeses is not recommended because they are difficult to digest, cause constipation, and are high in saturated fat and cholesterol.

Soy cheese may be bought at health markets and many grocery stores.

Soy milk. Soy milk is a good nondairy substitute for milk. Some people who don't like to drink it *do* enjoy it on cereals or in casseroles.

Soy milk now comes in vanilla and carob flavors as well as plain—perhaps there is a flavor you will like!

Sunflower seeds. Nothing can equal cashews when it comes to making the *creamiest* sauces, but sunflower seeds can be blended into very fine sauces, too. The advantages of sunflower seeds is that they are less expensive than cashews, and they can be used by people who are allergic to nuts.

Tofu. Tofu is soybean curd—a vegetarian source of high-quality, low-cost, cholesterol-free protein. It is low in fat, and a good source of calcium, phosphorus, iron, B vitamins, and protein. If you buy large quantities it can be frozen (this will change the texture), or kept refrigerated for one to two weeks (keep in an airtight container and change the water every day or so).

If you have trouble finding some of these ingredients and are unable to order them through your health food store, here are some sources you can try:

Ananda Products, 918 N. Broadway, Box 24125, Oklahoma City, OK 73124

Arrowhead Mills, Inc., P.O. Box 2059, 110 South Lawton St., Hereford, TX 79045

Cedarlane, 4928 Hollywood Blvd., Hollywood, CA 90027

El Molino Mills, 345 N. Baldwin Park Blvd., City of Industry, CA 91746

Food for Life, 3580 Pasadena Ave., Los Angeles, CA 90031

Garden of Eatin', 5300 Santa Monica Blvd., Hollywood, CA 90029

Health Valley Natural Foods, Montebello, CA 90640

Lifestream Natural Foods, Ltd., 1241 Vulcan Way, Richmond, B.C., Canada V6V 137

Soken Trading, Inc., 591 Redwood Hwy., Suite 2125, Mill Valley, CA 94941

Sovex Natural Foods, Box 310, Collegedale, TN 37315

Sun Ray, 570 N.E. 185th St., Miami, FL 35179

Tree of Life, 1750 Tree Blvd., St. Augustine, FL 32085

Epilogue

Jan welcomed you into this wellness adventure in the introduction. Now I want to close with some words of encouragement and some exciting news of the future.

For too long, America has been breaking its heart and soul with a life-style out of control. That doesn't have to continue. With extensive research now available on the health and longevity of Seventh-Day Adventists, many scientists view the Adventist life-style as a forecast of what Americans in general can experience as they embrace an all-encompassing approach to living better, slimmer, and longer.

You could be one of the first to blaze the way. In seven days—or seven weeks, however you decide to implement the program—you could be on your way to a new life, a new you. As you adopt the principles outlined in this book, a fundamental new concept will begin to shape your life: ideal weight, cholesterol management, and other signs of good health follow healthy living habits. And holding to the regimen only gets easier as you discover the rewards of pampering yourself with the truly best things in life.

It has been a joy working with Jan to make this health breakthrough available to you. After successfully adopting the Adventist-style approach to healthy living, Jan was quick to recognize its potential as a public service. It is our hope that this book will open the way to greater health and longevity for you, too, whatever your family and religious traditions, and that you will allow the principles to change your life as they have changed ours.

—Chris Rucker

References

The foundation of the healthful life-style of the Seventh-Day Adventist is a set of deeply held beliefs that have been tested by time and experience and do not stand or fall on evidence that may be presented in an isolated scientific study.

But these beliefs have also been tested by modern science. Though it is not the *basis* for the Adventist health principles, scientific research has provided evidence that overwhelmingly supports the soundness of these principles. And scientific techniques of statistical analysis have proved indisputably that Adventists have longer lives and greater freedom from disease than the general population. Adventists appreciate modern science for its ability to help us more fully understand the workings of the body, and to help give reasons that the health practices they have followed for a century and a half have been so successful.

In this spirit we offer you the following references for the information presented in this book. Some are studies as reported by the original researchers, some as reported in popular publications. Much current material (charts, statistics, and other information) was provided by John Scharffenberg, M.D., M.P.H.

Introduction

Seventh-Day Adventist longevity compared with that of the general population: Some figures reported by John Scharffenberg from ongoing Adventist Health Study. For other information, see J. Cook, "A church whose members have less cancer," *Saturday Evening Post,* March 1984, p. 42, and *Washington Post,* "The healthful lives of Adventists," November 22, 1988, p. 27.

Reduced risk of osteoporosis in Seventh-Day Adventists: A. Marsh, T. Sanchez, et al. "Critical bone density of adult lacto-ovo-vegetarian and omnivorous women." *J. Amer. Diet. Assoc.* 76 (1980): 148.

Low incidence of breast, prostate, pancreatic, and ovarian cancer in Seventh-Day Adventists: R. L. Phillips et al. Cancer in vegetarians, unpublished.

Low incidence of colon and rectal cancer in Seventh-Day Adventists: B. Liebman. "Are vegetarians healthier than the rest of us?" *Nutrition Action,* June 1983.

Comparative heart disease rates of Seventh-Day Adventists: R. L. Phillips, F. R. Lemon, W. L. Beeson, J. W. Kuzman. "Coronary heart disease mortality among Seventh-Day Adventists with differing dietary habits: A preliminary report." *Amer. J. Clin. Nutr.* 31 (1978): S-191–98.

Prophetic dietary statements of Ellen G. White: J. Cook, "A church whose members have less cancer," p. 40.

Chapter 1.   Principle No. 1 • Eat a Good Breakfast

Complex carbohydrates and lower incidence of heart disease: Senate Select Committee on Nutrition and Human Needs. *Dietary Goals for the United States.* Washington, D.C.: U.S. Printing Office, 1977, p. 17.

Attention problems of children who skip breakfast: J. Meer. "Breaking with breakfast." *Psychology Today,* August 1986, p. 6.

Breakfast and longevity: L. Berkman and L. Breslow. *Health and Ways of Living: The Alameda County Study.* New York: Oxford University Press, 1983, p. 88.

Satiety value of certain foods: Senate Select Committee. *Dietary Goals for the United States,* 1977, p. 4.

Obesity and food intake: F. Bellisle. "Obesity and food intake in children: Evidence for a role of metabolic and/or behavioral daily rhythms." *Appetite* 11, no. 2 (1988): 111–18.

NIH study and University of Minnesota study: J. Brody. *The Good Food Book.* New York: W. W. Norton, 1985, p. 189.

Chapter 2.   Principle No. 2 • Cut Out Empty and Refined Calories

Dental caries and use of sugar: Garn, Cole, Solomon, and Schaefer. "Relationships between sugar foods and the DMFT in 1968–1970." *Ecology of Food and Nutrition* 9 (1980): 135–38.

Diabetes and use of sugar: Campbell, Batchelor, and Goldberg. "Sugar intake and diabetes." *J. Amer. Diet. Assoc.* 50 (1967): 319.

Depressed immune response and use of sugar: Kijak, Foust, and Steinman. "Relationship of blood sugar level and leukocytic phagocytosis." *J. Southern California State Dental Association* 32 (1964): 349–51.

Hypoglycemia and use of sugar: R. Bolton. *Aggression in Quolla Society.* Champaign, Ill.: Garland Press, 1978.

Hypoglycemia and use of sugar: Sanders, Hofeldt, Kirk, and Levin. "Refined carbohydrate as a contributing factor in reactive hypoglycemia." *Southern Medical Journal* 75 (1982): 1072.

Triglyceride and cholesterol levels and use of sugar: L. Walton, J. Walton, and J. Scharffenberg. *Six Extra Years.* Santa Barbara, Calif.: Woodbridge Press, 1988, p. 18.

Chapter 3.   Principle No. 3 • Increase Fruits and Vegetables

Chronic degenerative diseases and consumption of vegetables: American Dietetic Association. Position paper on the vegetarian approach to eating. *J. Amer. Diet. Assoc.* 77 (1980): 61–70.

Vegetable consumption and avoidance of cancer: J. D. Potter. "Dietary fiber, vegetables, and cancer." *Journal of Nutrition* 118 (1988): 1591–92.

Calories and foods of low-caloric density: O. W. Wooley. "Long-term food regulation in the obese." *Psychosomatic Medicine* 33 (1971): 436–44.

Fiber as a vehicle to remove excess bile acids: E. L. Wynder. "Dietary environment and cancer." *J. Amer. Diet. Assoc.* 71 (1977): 385–92.

Fiber sources that lower serum cholesterol: J. W. Anderson. "Taking oat bran to heart (lowering cholesterol)," *Saturday Evening Post,* July/August 1989, p. 18.

Chapter 4.   Principle No. 4 • Go Low on Fat

General information on atherosclerosis: G. Wilson, M.D. "Atherosclerosis." Hartland Health Center, Rapidan, Va., 1986. Audiocassette.

Blood cholesterol and heart disease: Consensus Conference on "Lowering blood cholesterol to prevent heart disease." *J. Amer. Med. Assoc.* 253 (1985): 2080–97.

Vegetarian nutrition: M. G. Hardinge and F. J. Stare. "Nutritional studies of vegetarians: Nutritional, physical and laboratory studies." *Amer. J. Clin. Nutr.* 2 (1954): 73–82.

Vegetarian nutrition: "What doctors are learning from vegetarians." *Prevention* 38 (1986): 115.

Vegetarian diet: American Dietetic Association. Position paper on the vegetarian approach to eating. *J. Amer. Diet. Assoc.* 77 (1980): 61–70.

Manufacture of B_{12} in small intestine: "Contributions of microflora of the small intestine to vitamine B_{12} nutriture of man." *Nutr. Rev.* 38 (1980): 274–75.

Chapter 5.   Principle No. 5 • The Fast

Weight loss on two meals a day: D. A. Seaton and L. J. P. Duncan. "Treatment of 'refractory obesity' with a diet of two meals per day." *The Lancet,* September 19, 1964, p. 613.

Snacking between meals as a cause of tooth decay: B. J. Martin and J. S. Stewart. "The relationship between breakfast and snacking and the incidence of dental caries." *Oral Health* 73, no. 11 (1983): 65–66.

Quotation of Ellen G. White: Counsels on Diet and Foods (Letter 73, 1896). Washington, D.C.: Review and Herald Publishing Association, 1938, p. 90.

Chapter 6.   Principle No. 6 • Exercise

Exercise frequency statistic: American Sports Data, Inc., a Westchester, N.Y.–based firm that specializes in health and leisure statistics.

The preventive and therapeutic effects of exercise with regards to diabetes: "NIH consensus panel concludes that weight reduction and exercise are best therapy for people with type 2 diabetes," *Chicago Tribune,* January 18, 1987, section 5, p. 5, and "Benefits of exercise for diabetics," *New York Times,* Personal Health (Jane Brody), March 31, 1988, section B, p. 12.

The benefits of exercise in a cholesterol-control program: "Life in the slow lane" (research by Walker Buckalew), *Prevention* 39 (1987): 8.

Exercise and longevity: "Exercise and longevity: A little goes a long way." *New York Times,* November 3, 1989, section A, p. 1.

Benefits of exercise, including raising of HDL levels and protection from osteoporosis and diseases of the heart and blood levels: K. Cooper, *The Aerobics Program for Total Well-Being,* New York: M. Evans and Co., 1982.

Exercise, aging, and cancer: "Sweat cure: Exercise may prevent cancer" (study by R. E. Frisch). *Time,* February 29, 1988, p. 68.

Beneficial effects of exercise on sleep and productivity: "Wellness plan —perk that pays off." *Atlanta Journal,* June 3, 1989, section XJ, p. 11.

Chapter 7.   Program Your Mind for Success

T. L. Nichols. *Esoteric Anthropology.* New York: Stringer and Townsend, 1853.

W. Whitman. *The Complete Poetry and Prose of Walt Whitman (Deathbed Edition),* Vol. 2. New York: Garden City Books, 1954, p. 513.

J. Allen. "As a Man Thinketh." New York: T. Y. Crowell, 1913.

P. A. Stitt. *Fighting the Food Giants.* Natural Press, 1980.

A. Ries. *Positioning: The Battle for Your Mind.* New York: Warner Books, 1986.

L. Berkowitz. "The effects of observing violence." *Scientific American* 210, no. 2 (1964): 35.

216

Weight-Loss Record

Enter your current weight at the top of the column preceding Week 1. Weigh yourself weekly, entering your weight in that week's column, an appropriate number of spaces below your starting weight (1 pound = 1 space). Over the weeks, you'll be making a graph of your weight loss.

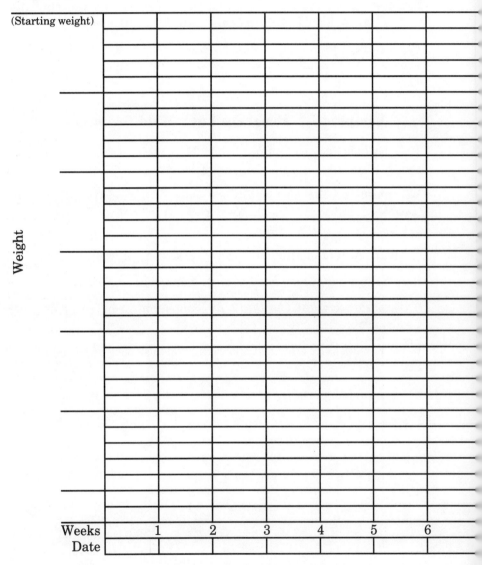

8	9	10	11	12	13	14	15	16	17

Desirable Weights According to Frame
at Ages 25 and Over
Weight in Pounds in Indoor Clothing

Height Without Shoes	Small Frame	Medium Frame	Large Frame
Men			
5'2"	115–123	121–133	129–144
4"	121–129	127–139	135–152
6"	128–137	134–147	142–161
8"	136–145	142–156	151–170
10"	144–154	150–165	159–179
6'0"	152–162	158–175	168–189
2"	160–171	167–185	178–199
4"	168–179	177–195	187–209
Women			
4'10"	96–104	101–113	109–125
5'0"	102–110	107–119	115–131
2"	108–116	113–126	121–138
4"	114–123	120–135	129–146
6"	122–131	128–143	137–154
8"	130–140	136–151	145–163
10"	138–148	144–159	153–173

Adapted from Metropolitan Life Insurance Company Tables

Index

About the Authors

CHRISTINE J. RUCKER is a health educator who for more than twenty years has been teaching the benefits of healthful living to individuals and organizations. She has directed community health education services and has consulted for community and teaching hospitals. She is the founder of Abundant Life Associates, a consulting group that conducts life-style management classes and seminars on smoking cessation, weight and nutrition management, and stress management. (For further information on available seminars, write to Abundant Life Associates, P.O. Box 540163, Orlando, FL 32854-0163.) A frequent guest speaker for churches and public health agencies, she has conducted cooking schools and seminars throughout the United States and promotes healthy life-style habits on television and radio. She is married to a hospital and health-care administrator and has three children.

JAN HOFFMAN is a writer and artist specializing in portraiture and watercolor. After experiencing the benefits of the Adventist approach to weight control and health in Chris Rucker's classes, she wanted to help spread the word. She lives in Nashville, Tennessee, with her two daughters.